THE DIRTY RESET COOKBOOK

— 30 Days. My Way. —

REAL FOOD FOR REAL LIFE

30 DAYS OF DINNERS THAT FIT YOUR LIFE + EXTRAS

WENDY LITTRELL

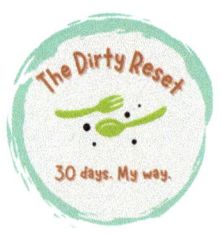 | # THE DIRTY RESET™

Copyright © 2025 by Wendy Littrell

All rights reserved. No part of this publication may be reproduced, distributed, or transmitted in any form or by any means, including photocopying, recording, or other electronic or mechanical methods, without the prior written permission of the author, except in the case of brief quotations used in critical reviews or certain other noncommercial uses permitted by copyright law.

ISBN: 979-8-218-68600-0
Published by: The Dirty Reset™
Printed in the United States of America
Website: www.thedirtyreset.com

Trademark Notice
The Dirty Reset™ is a trademark of Wendy Littrell. Use of this name and brand without permission is strictly prohibited.

Disclaimer
This book is an independent work based on the author's personal experience. It is not affiliated with or endorsed by any external organization. Recipes in *The Dirty Reset™ Cookbook* have not been professionally tested in a lab kitchen; they were developed, prepared, and refined in a home setting. All measurements and ingredients are provided to the best of the author's ability. Readers are encouraged to use their own discretion when adapting or substituting ingredients.

The recipes and content in this book are intended for informational and inspirational purposes only. The author does not provide medical or nutritional advice, and this book is not a substitute for professional guidance. Always consult a qualified health provider with any questions regarding your dietary needs or a medical condition.

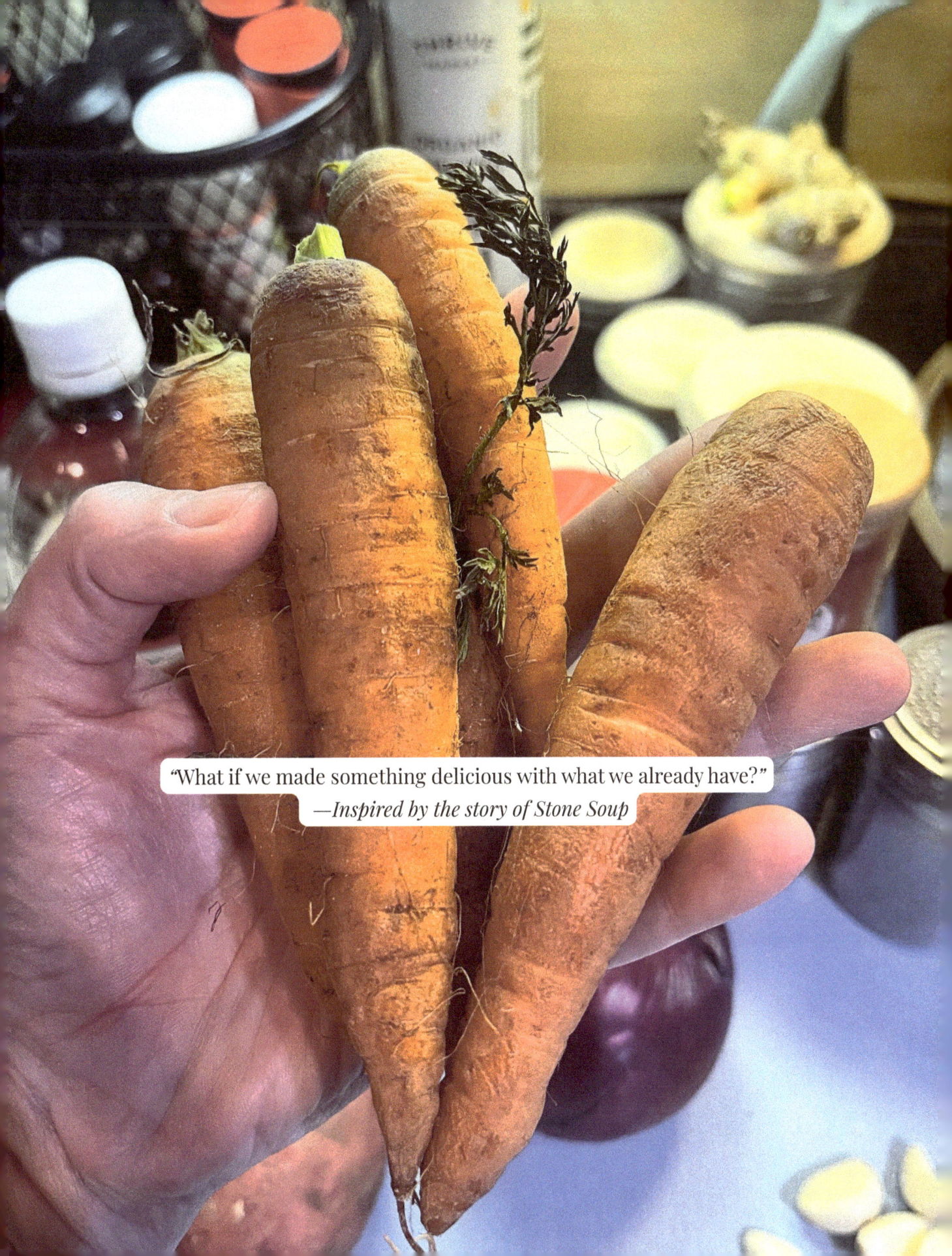

"What if we made something delicious with what we already have?"
—*Inspired by the story of Stone Soup*

DEDICATION

To my husband—

You didn't just cheer me on, you did it with me.

Every step, every taste test, every moment, you were there.

Thank you for making this something we shared.

Thank you for making this something we built together.

I loved doing this with you.

CONTENTS

My Dirty Reset Story..1
How to Use This Cookbook..2
Putting It All Together..3
The Dirty Reset: 30-Day Dinner Calendar....................................5
The Dirty Reset: Day-by-Day Dinners...9
Dirty Extras..43
Dirty Side Dishes..49
The Dirty Sauce: Sauces & Condiments.....................................59
Dirty Sweets...71
What About Breakfast & Lunch?..79
After The Dirty Reset..81
Acknowledgments..83
About the Author...85

MY DIRTY RESET STORY

Welcome to The Dirty Reset™! Like a lot of people, I struggled to find a way of eating that felt good without obsessing over perfection. I wanted meals that actually fit my real life, things I could cook, enjoy, and keep coming back to without overthinking every bite.

The Dirty Reset started as my own experiment with 30 days of simple, whole-food meals, but with flexibility, comfort, and no guilt. I didn't want to be hungry, and I definitely didn't want to count calories. Along the way, I realized that what matters most isn't following strict rules, it's showing up for yourself, doing your best, and letting that be enough.

This cookbook is a reflection of that experience, built from the real dinners I cooked, tasted, and shared on my YouTube channel, The Dirty Reset. There, I post quick shorts with simple visual steps designed to spark ideas and show how approachable these meals can be. My goal is to give you inspiration to feed yourself well in a way that works for you.

In The Dirty Reset, every recipe is naturally gluten-free, dairy-free, soy-free, and free from refined sugar. This isn't because dairy, soy, or grains can't be whole foods. These recipes just naturally take shape without them. Things like coconut aminos, avocado oil, and ghee are staples in my kitchen and might be new to you, but they are easy to find and worth keeping on hand.

So here I am, just a mom with a camera at my kitchen counter, sharing what worked for me and hoping it inspires you to find what works for you, too.

Wendy

HOW TO USE THIS COOKBOOK

The Dirty Reset™ is real food with real-life flexibility.
No tracking, no guilt, just meals that taste good and keep you going.

Inside, you'll find 30 days of simple dinners plus Dirty Extras for sauces, sweets, and sides. Follow the meals in order or jump around based on what sounds good. No perfection required, just comfort food, one meal at a time.

During this stretch, you'll focus on real ingredients and set aside the ultra-processed stuff. That means no refined sugars, refined grains, or unpronounceable mystery ingredients. The recipes also naturally leave out dairy, soy, legumes, and alcohol, not because you have to, but because it's worth noticing how your body feels with fewer of the extras and more of the foods that keep things simple and satisfying.

When something needs a little sweetness, I stick with real fruit, sometimes blended into the recipe and sometimes added on the side. For baking or sauces, I love using dates, date syrup, or date sugar straight from nature, because they are whole-food options instead of processed sugars like white sugar or corn syrup.

How to Start your Dirty Reset:
1. Pick a dinner—start at Day 1 or skip around using the provided calendar.
2. No rules on portions or servings. Just make the food.
3. Missing something? Swap it. Add stuff. Make it yours.
4. Want extras? Grab a side or sauce from the Dirty Extras.
5. Need to pause or repeat a day? Go for it. This isn't a challenge, it's dinner.

Use this book like a flexible tool, not a rulebook, and build a way of eating you actually want to come back to. Spend 30 days with these recipes, or simply use them when you need inspiration. This isn't a promise or a magic fix. It is a stretch of simple recipes that can help nourish your body, your energy, and your habits. Whether you notice more comfort in your body or more ease in your kitchen, The Dirty Reset is here to help you find what works for you.

PUTTING IT ALL TOGETHER

Here's the basic formula:
Protein + Veggies + Flavor + Comfort
- Protein: Chicken, beef, fish, shrimp, eggs, or plant-based options
- Veggies: Roasted, sautéed, raw, or blended into sauces
- Flavor Booster: Garlic, coconut aminos, herbs, vinegar, sauces, seasoning blends
- Comfort Element: Potatoes, roasted sweet potatoes or squash, creamy risotto, broth, fried egg, grain-free noodles, plantain chips

Think skillet meals, sheet pans, stews, or bowls, all made from whole ingredients you recognize. You can follow the plan or simply cook what works for your week. Go 30 days straight or pick and choose. Don't have something? Swap it.

Need to round out a meal? Here's how:
Some meals in this cookbook are packed with veggies and protein, while others (like crab legs) are more of a fun main dish that's just waiting for something on the side. If dinner feels a little light or one-note, it's easy to round it out. Just build a plate that feels good to you.

Easy ways to round out a meal:
- Side salad with The Dirty Reset Sweet Balsamic Salad Dressing
- Roasted or sautéed vegetables
- Mashed or baked potatoes
- A fruit bowl or sliced avocado
- Soup or broth to start

Build meals that feel good, because this is about eating better, not stressing more. These 30 days are a starting point to help shift the way you eat toward something more grounded, more satisfying, and more doable long-term. No extremes. Just real food that works in real life.

THE DIRTY RESET™ 30-DAY DINNER CALENDAR

30 days. My way.

thedirtyreset.com | @thedirtyreset

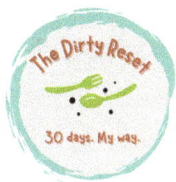

DAY 1	DAY 2	DAY 3	DAY 4	DAY 5
Coconut Chicken Skillet	Shepherd's Pie	Oven-Baked Chicken	Weeknight Beef Stew	Simple Ramen Bowl
DAY 6	**DAY 7**	**DAY 8**	**DAY 9**	**DAY 10**
Chicken Salad	Pan-Fried Tilapia	Chicken & Butternut Bake	Lemon Garlic Salmon	Baked Chicken Wings
DAY 11	**DAY 12**	**DAY 13**	**DAY 14**	**DAY 15**
Crab Legs Night	Steak & Baked Potatoes	Fresh Chopped Salad	Sweet Mustard Meatloaf	One-Pan Dirty Thighs
DAY 16	**DAY 17**	**DAY 18**	**DAY 19**	**DAY 20**
Bolognese Meat Sauce	Slow-Cooked Pulled Pork	Sausage & Veggie Skillet	Hearty Chili	Korean Lettuce Cups
DAY 21	**DAY 22**	**DAY 23**	**DAY 24**	**DAY 25**
Orange Chicken & Broccoli	Fish Chowder	Egg Roll Bowl	Chicken Soup	Cider-Kissed Pork Chops
DAY 26	**DAY 27**	**DAY 28**	**DAY 29**	**DAY 30**
Seafood Night	Curry & Mashed Potatoes	Slow-Baked Ribs	Sweet & Spicy Mango Shrimp	One-Pan Dirty Hash

This calendar shows the dinners cooked during the 30-day Dirty Reset. Use it as inspiration, a starting point, or follow it day by day, whatever fits your life. No rules, no tracking. Just real food, one good meal at a time. The recipes for every meal are just ahead.

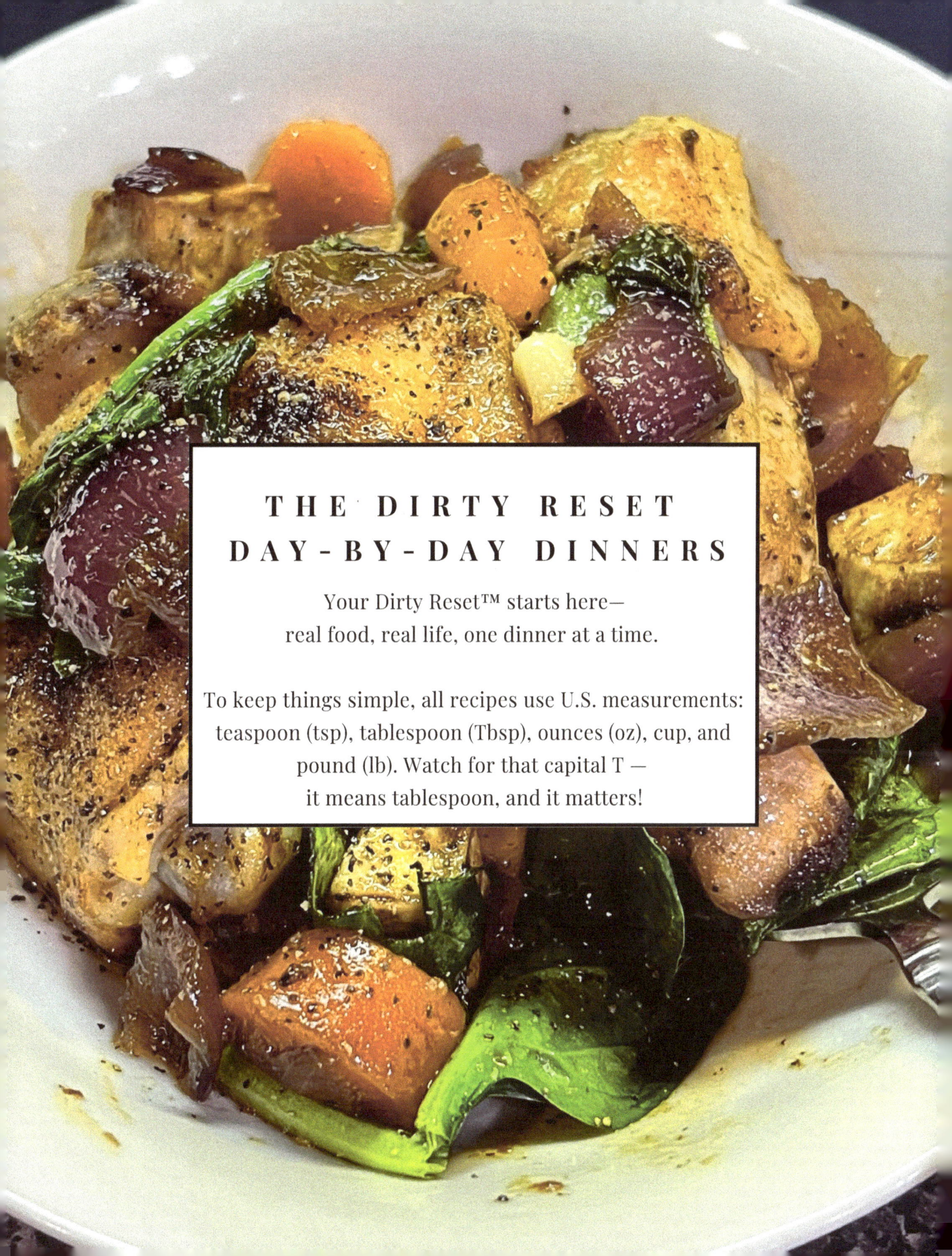

THE DIRTY RESET
DAY-BY-DAY DINNERS

Your Dirty Reset™ starts here—
real food, real life, one dinner at a time.

To keep things simple, all recipes use U.S. measurements:
teaspoon (tsp), tablespoon (Tbsp), ounces (oz), cup, and
pound (lb). Watch for that capital T —
it means tablespoon, and it matters!

The Dirty Reset
Day-by-Day Dinners

- Day 1: Coconut Chicken Skillet
- Day 2: Shepherd's Pie
- Day 3: Oven-Baked Chicken
- Day 4: Weeknight Beef Stew
- Day 5: Simple Ramen Bowl
- Day 6: Chicken Salad
- Day 7: Pan-Fried Tilapia
- Day 8: Chicken & Butternut Bake
- Day 9: Lemon Garlic Salmon
- Day 10: Baked Chicken Wings
- Day 11: Crab Legs Night
- Day 12: Steak & Baked Potatoes
- Day 13: Fresh Chopped Salad
- Day 14: Sweet Mustard Meatloaf
- Day 15: One-Pan Dirty Thighs
- Day 16: Bolognese Meat Sauce
- Day 17: Slow-Cooked Pulled Pork
- Day 18: Sausage & Veggie Skillet
- Day 19: Hearty Chili
- Day 20: Korean Lettuce Cups
- Day 21: Orange Chicken & Broccoli
- Day 22: Fish Chowder
- Day 23: Egg Roll Bowl
- Day 24: Chicken Soup
- Day 25: Cider-Kissed Pork Chops
- Day 26: Seafood Night
- Day 27: Curry & Mashed Potatoes
- Day 28: Slow-Baked Ribs
- Day 29: Sweet & Spicy Mango Shrimp
- Day 30: One-Pan Dirty Hash

DAY 1
COCONUT CHICKEN SKILLET

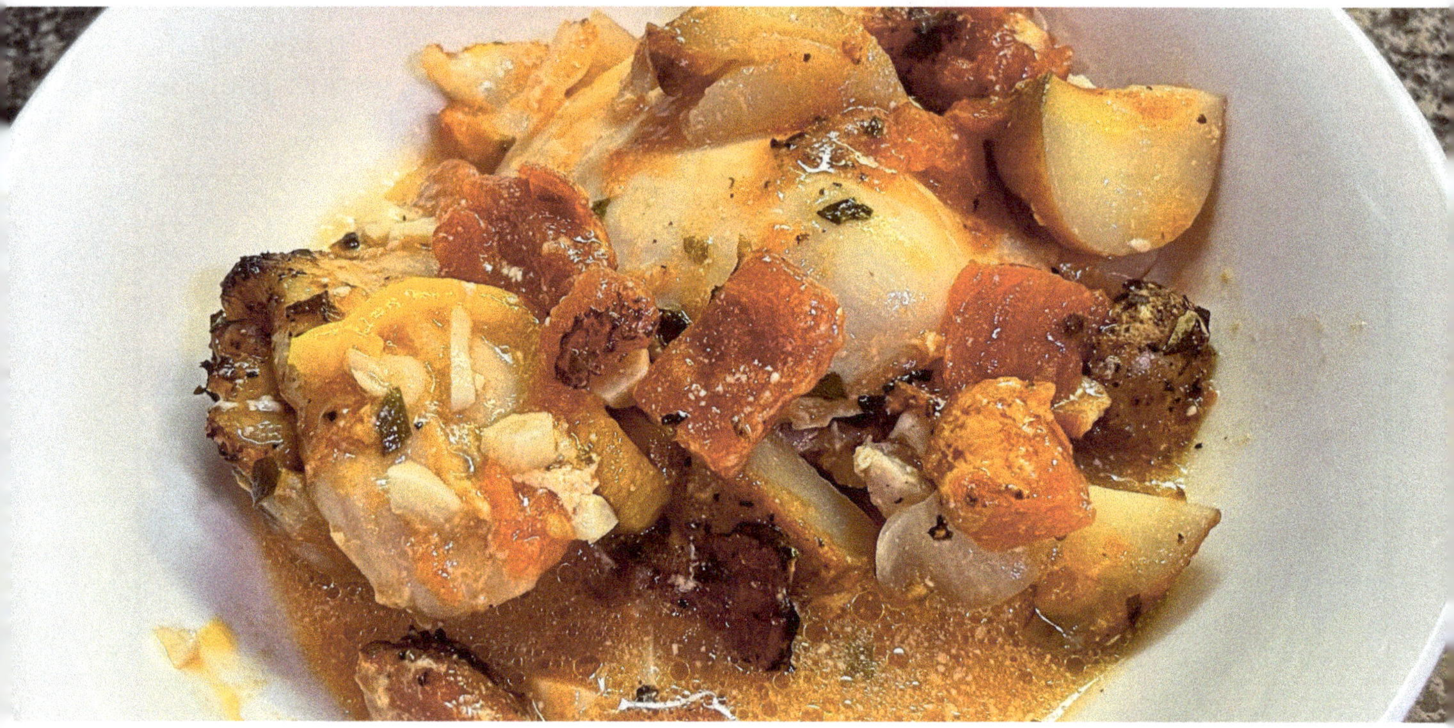

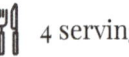 4 servings 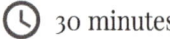 30 minutes

INGREDIENTS

- 2 Tbsp avocado or olive oil
- 4–6 boneless, skinless chicken breasts
- Salt & pepper to taste
- 1 medium onion, sliced
- 3 cloves garlic, minced
- 1 can (14.5 oz) fire-roasted diced tomatoes
- 1 can (13.5 oz) full-fat coconut milk
- 1 Tbsp coconut aminos
- 1 Tbsp lime juice
- Optional: fresh cilantro or lime wedges for serving

DIRECTIONS

1. Preheat oven to 375°F.
2. Heat oil in a large oven-safe skillet over medium-high heat.
3. Season chicken breasts with salt and pepper.
4. Sear chicken 3–4 minutes per side until golden. Remove and set aside.
5. In the same skillet, sauté onion until soft. Add garlic and cook 1 more minute.
6. Stir in the fire-roasted diced tomatoes and let them simmer for 2–3 minutes.
7. Add coconut milk, coconut aminos, and lime juice. Bring to a simmer.
8. Return chicken to the skillet. Spoon sauce over the top.
9. Transfer skillet to oven and bake 20–25 minutes until chicken is cooked through or until it reaches an internal temperature of 165°F.
10. Garnish with cilantro or lime wedges if desired before serving.

The coconut-tomato sauce makes this a repeat-worthy one-pan dinner. Spoon extra sauce over veggies or save it for tomorrow's lunch.

DAY 2
SHEPHERD'S PIE

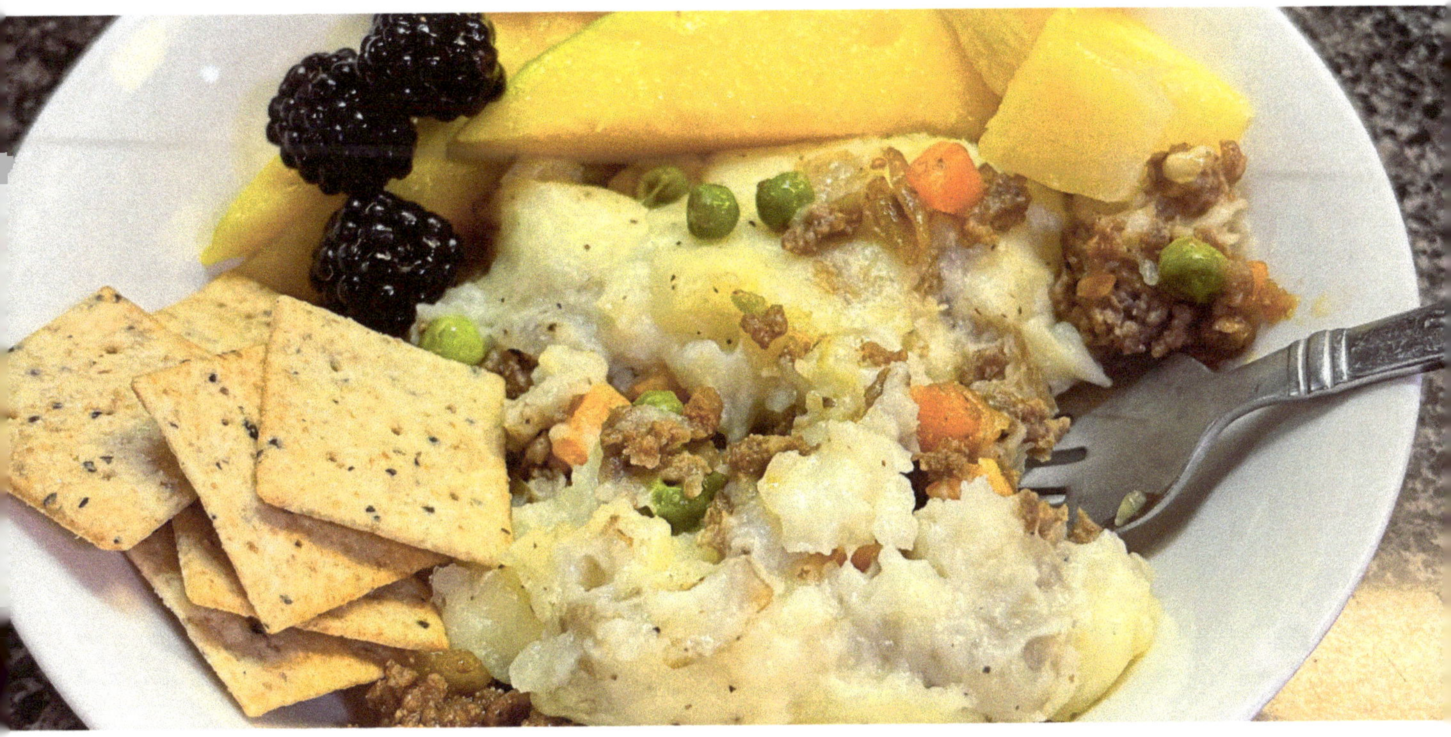

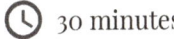 4 servings 30 minutes

INGREDIENTS

- Avocado or olive oil
- 1 lb ground beef
- Salt & pepper to taste
- 1 medium onion, diced
- 2 cloves garlic, minced
- 2 Tbsp tomato paste
- 1 Tbsp coconut aminos
- 1 tsp dried thyme
- 1 tsp dried oregano
- ½ tsp garlic powder
- ½ tsp onion powder
- 2 cups mixed vegetables
- 4 cups The Dirty Reset™ Mashed Potatoes (see Dirty Side Dishes section for recipe)

DIRECTIONS

1. Preheat oven to 400°F.
2. In a large oven-safe skillet, cook the ground beef over medium heat until browned. If using lean ground beef, add a drizzle of oil first. Drain excess fat if needed; if your beef is higher in fat, you may not need extra oil.
3. Add ground beef, season with salt and pepper, and cook until browned. Drain excess fat if necessary.
4. Add diced onion and cook until softened. Stir in minced garlic and cook for 1 more minute.
5. Stir in tomato paste, coconut aminos, thyme, oregano, garlic powder, and onion powder. Mix well.
6. Add mixed vegetables and cook until just tender. Adjust seasoning as needed.
7. Spread mashed potatoes evenly over the beef mixture right in the oven-safe skillet.
8. Transfer the skillet to the oven and bake for 20–25 minutes, until the top is lightly golden. Let cool slightly before serving.

> This skillet version saves time and dishes. Make extra mashed potatoes — they freeze great and reheat like a dream.

DAY 3
OVEN-BAKED CHICKEN

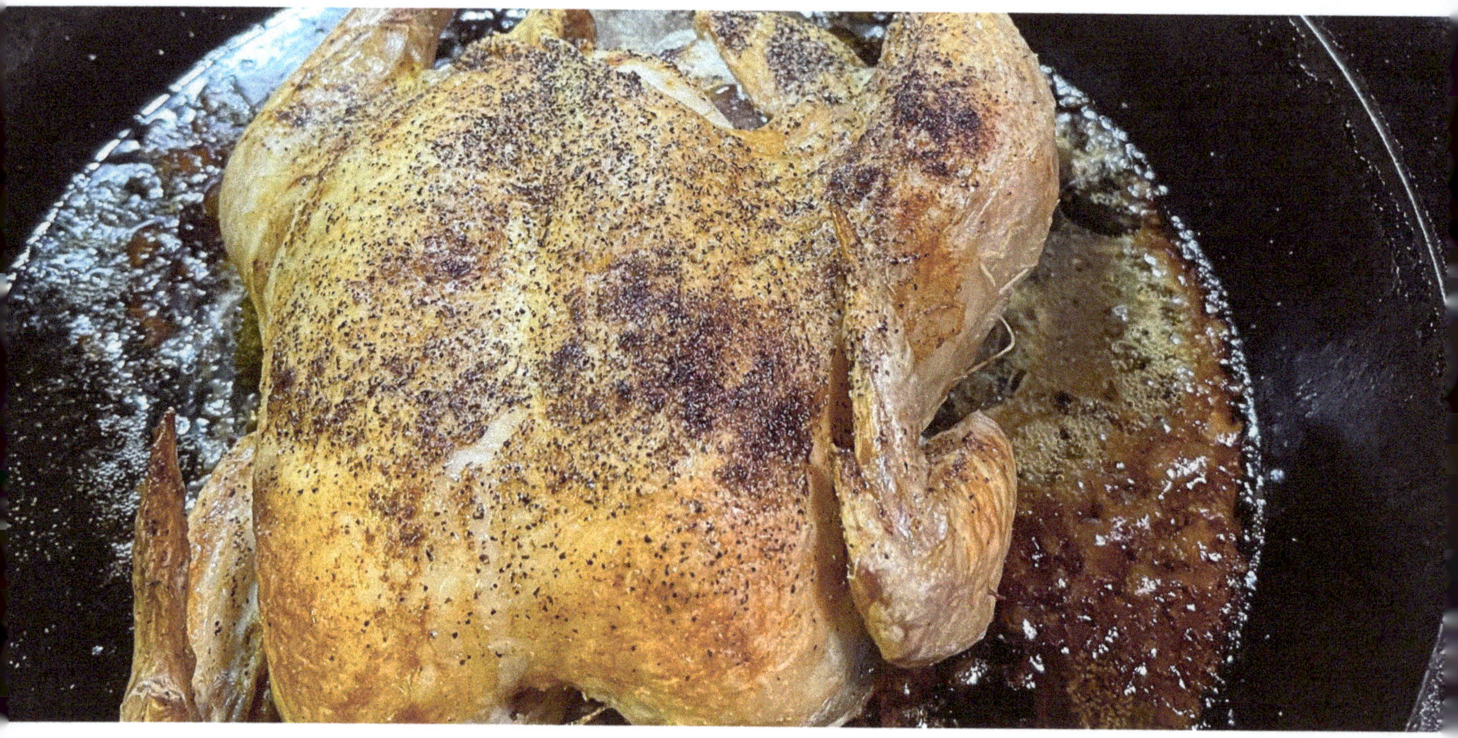

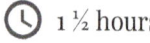

 4 servings   🕐 1 ½ hours

INGREDIENTS

- 1 whole chicken (about 4-6 lbs)
- 2-3 Tbsp avocado or olive oil (or ghee)
- 2 tsp garlic powder
- 2 tsp onion powder
- 1 tsp paprika
- 1 tsp dried oregano
- Salt & pepper to taste
- Optional: lemon halves, garlic cloves, and fresh herbs for stuffing the cavity

DIRECTIONS

1. Preheat oven to 400°F. Pat the chicken dry with paper towels.
2. Rub oil or ghee over the entire chicken. For extra flavor and moisture, work some under the skin, especially over the breast.
3. Mix garlic powder, onion powder, paprika, oregano, salt, and pepper in a small bowl. Rub the seasoning mix all over the chicken, inside and out.
4. Optional: stuff the cavity with lemon halves, garlic cloves, and fresh herbs if desired.
5. Place the chicken breast-side up in a roasting pan, with the wings tucked underneath.
6. Roast for about 1 hour 15 minutes to 1 hour 30 minutes, or until the internal temperature reaches 165°F in the thickest part of the thigh.
7. Let rest 10 minutes before carving.

Roast once, eat twice — save leftover meat for salads, soups, or skillet meals.
Don't toss the bones; they make rich homemade broth (see Dirty Extras section for recipe).

DAY 4
WEEKNIGHT BEEF STEW

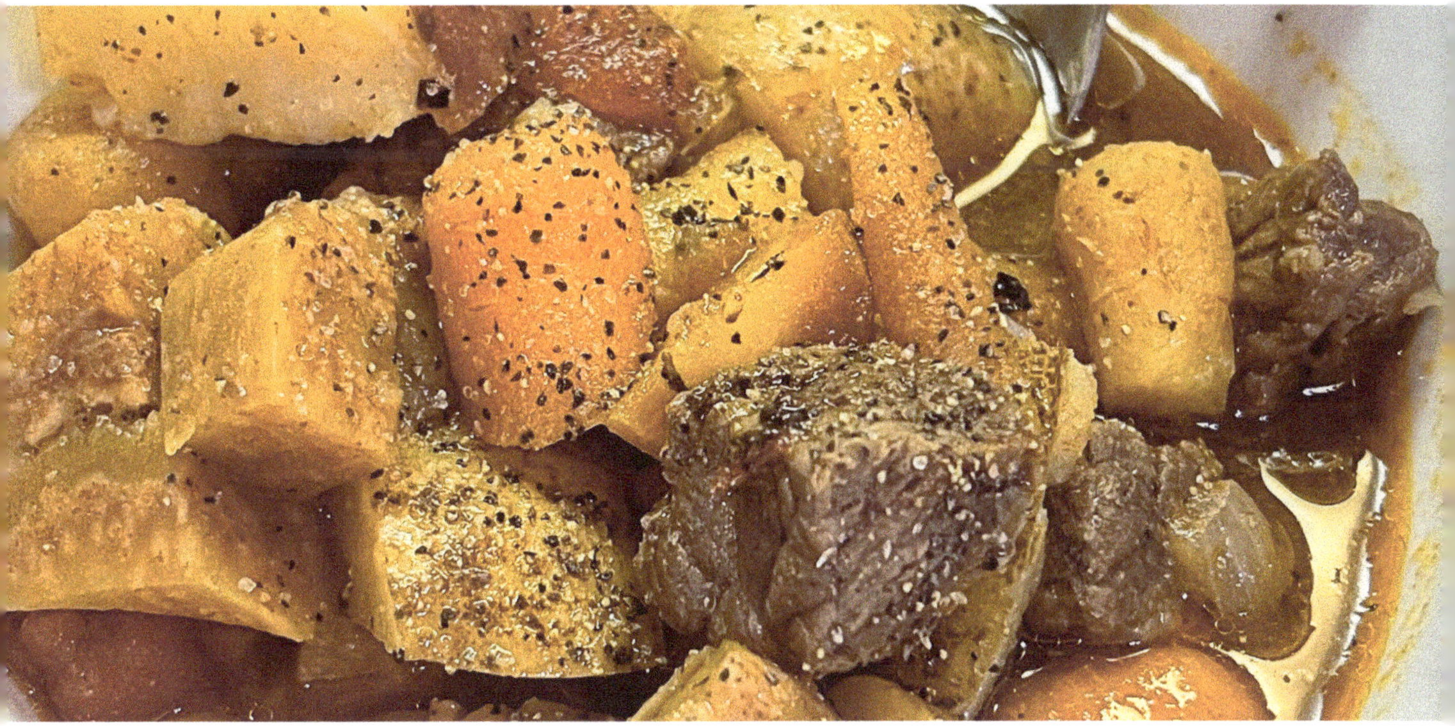

 4 servings 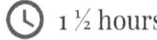 1 ½ hours

INGREDIENTS

- Avocado or olive oil
- 1.5 to 2 lbs beef round steak or stew meat, cut into chunks
- 1 medium onion, chopped
- 2–3 cloves garlic, minced
- 3 medium carrots, sliced
- 2 stalks celery, chopped
- 1 can (14.5 oz) diced tomatoes
- 4 cups beef broth
- 2 Tbsp coconut aminos
- 1 tsp garlic powder
- 1 tsp onion powder
- 1 tsp smoked paprika
- ½ tsp dried thyme
- Salt & pepper to taste
- 2 green plantains or potatoes, peeled and diced
- 1 ½ Tbsp tapioca flour
- 3 Tbsp cool water
- Optional: chopped parsley for garnish

DIRECTIONS

1. Heat a bit of oil in a large pot or Dutch oven over medium-high heat. Add beef chunks and brown on all sides. Remove and set aside.
2. In the same pot, add onion, garlic, carrots, and celery. Cook for 3-4 minutes until slightly softened.
3. Return the beef to the pot. Stir in diced tomatoes, beef broth, coconut aminos, garlic powder, onion powder, smoked paprika, thyme, salt, and pepper.
4. Bring to a boil, then reduce heat and simmer covered for about 1 hour, stirring occasionally.
5. Add diced plantains or potatoes and continue to simmer for another 20-30 minutes, until beef is tender and plantains are soft.
6. Once stew is fully cooked, lower the heat to a gentle simmer. Whisk tapioca flour with cool water until completely smooth. Slowly stir into stew while mixing well. Simmer for 1-2 minutes until thickened to your liking. For extra body, mash a few chunks of cooked plantain, potato, or carrot into the pot before adding the slurry.
7. Taste and adjust seasoning if needed. Garnish with chopped parsley if desired and serve hot.

Short on time? This stew works great in a pressure cooker like the Ninja Foodi. Just reduce the liquid slightly and cook on high for about 35 minutes.

DAY 5
SIMPLE RAMEN BOWL

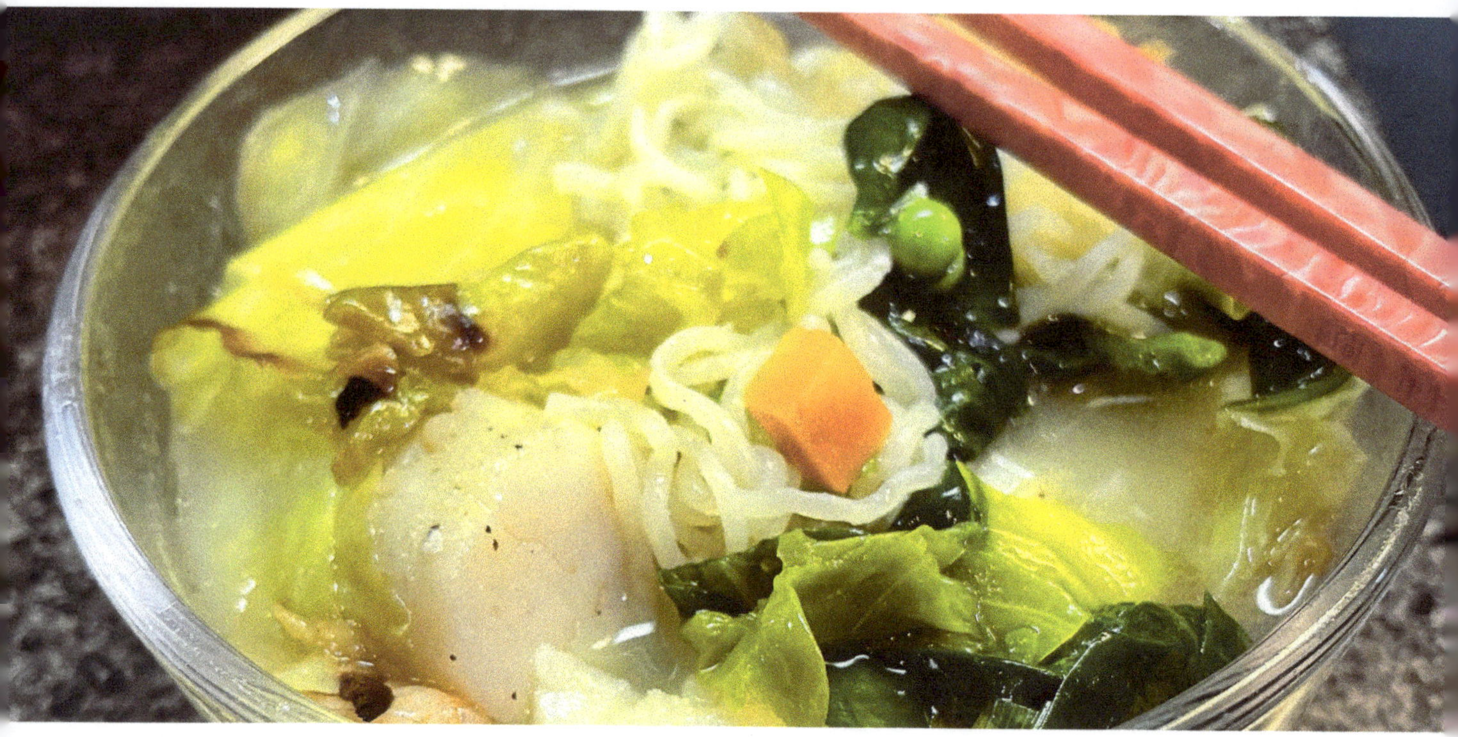

 4 servings 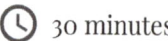 30 minutes

INGREDIENTS

- 8 cups chicken or beef broth
- 3 Tbsp sesame oil
- 4-5 cloves garlic, chopped
- 2-inch piece fresh ginger, chopped
- Salt & pepper to taste
- 3-4 scallions, chopped (white and green parts separated)
- 3 to 4 cups chopped or shredded cabbage
- Avocado or olive oil (for frying cabbage)
- Noodles: zucchini spirals (zoodles) or shirataki noodles
- 2 cups mixed vegetables
- 1 cup mushrooms, sliced
- 2 to 3 cups fresh spinach
- 3-4 cups cooked chicken or any cooked meat of choice (optional)

DIRECTIONS

1. In a stockpot, heat the broth over medium-high heat. Add sesame oil, garlic, ginger, salt, pepper, and the white parts of the scallions.
2. Bring to a boil and simmer for about 7-10 minutes to infuse the broth with flavor.
3. Meanwhile, salt the chopped cabbage, then fry it in a skillet with oil until softened. Set aside for serving.
4. If using zucchini spirals or shirataki noodles, prepare them according to package instructions (usually a quick rinse and light sauté if needed).
5. Once the broth is ready, add the mixed vegetables and mushrooms. Simmer for 3-4 minutes.
6. Add fresh spinach last and cook just until wilted (about 30 seconds to 1 minute). Remove from heat.
7. To serve, place cooked noodles, optional cooked meat, and fried cabbage into bowls. Ladle hot broth and vegetables over the top.
8. Garnish with the green parts of the scallions. Serve hot.

Zucchini noodles keep this light, but shirataki makes it feel like takeout.
Add a soft-boiled egg on top for a cozy upgrade.

DAY 6
CHICKEN SALAD

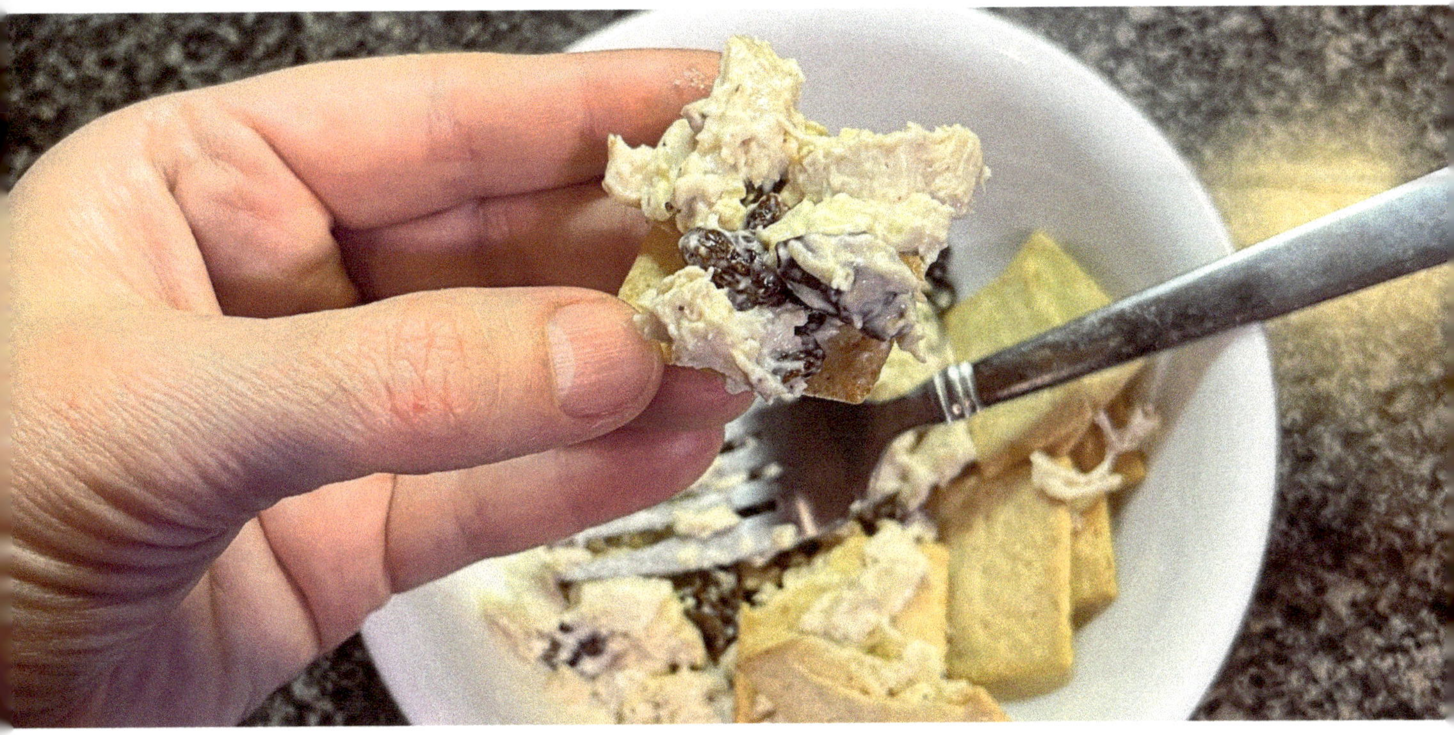

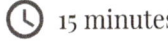 4 servings   15 minutes

INGREDIENTS

- 2 to 3 cups cooked chicken, chopped
- 1 to 2 Tbsp onion, minced
- 1 rib celery, minced
- 1–2 tsp lemon juice
- Salt & pepper to taste
- 1 tsp coconut aminos
- 1 tsp Dijon mustard (optional)
- ½ to 1 cup avocado mayo
- ½ to ¾ cup seedless grapes, chopped (or ¼ cup raisins)
- ¼ tsp celery seed

DIRECTIONS

1. In a large bowl, combine the chicken, onion, celery, lemon juice, salt, pepper, coconut aminos, and Dijon if using. Stir in the avocado mayo at the end so you can adjust the amount as needed.
2. Stir until well mixed. Gently fold in grapes or raisins.
3. Sprinkle top with celery seed. Taste and adjust seasoning if needed.
4. Serve chilled in lettuce cups or straight from the bowl.

This fast and flexible creamy chicken salad works with whatever chicken you have, whether roasted, canned, or from your Oven-Baked Chicken (Day 3 recipe).

Day 7
Pan-Fried Tilapia

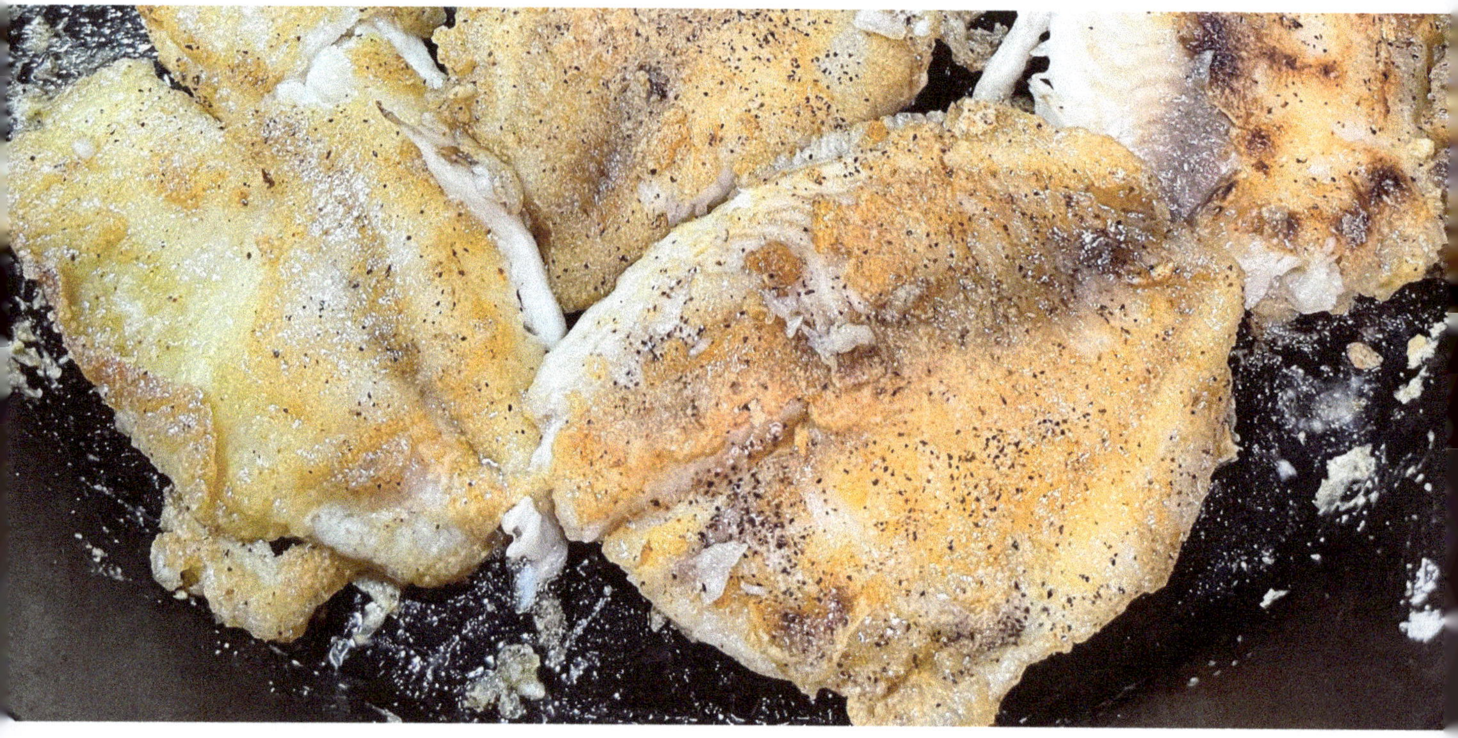

 4 servings 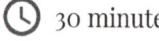 30 minutes

INGREDIENTS

- 1 egg
- 2 Tbsp coconut aminos
- ½ cup tapioca flour
- 1 tsp smoked paprika
- ½ tsp garlic powder
- ½ tsp onion powder
- Salt & pepper to taste
- 4 tilapia fillets (or other white fish such as catfish, swai, cod, or haddock), thawed if frozen
- Avocado oil for frying
- Lemon wedges, for serving

DIRECTIONS

1. In a shallow bowl, whisk the egg with coconut aminos.
2. In another shallow dish, combine tapioca flour, smoked paprika, garlic powder, onion powder, salt, and pepper.
3. Pat tilapia fillets dry. Dip each fillet first in the egg wash, then dredge in the flour mixture until well coated.
4. Heat about ¼ inch of oil in a skillet over medium heat.
5. Fry tilapia 2–3 minutes per side, until golden and crispy.
6. Drain on paper towels and serve with lemon wedges.

Tapioca flour gives that perfect crisp without the grain.
Serve with The Dirty Reset™ Tartar Sauce for extra kick (see The Dirty Sauce section for recipe).

Day 8
CHICKEN & BUTTERNUT BAKE

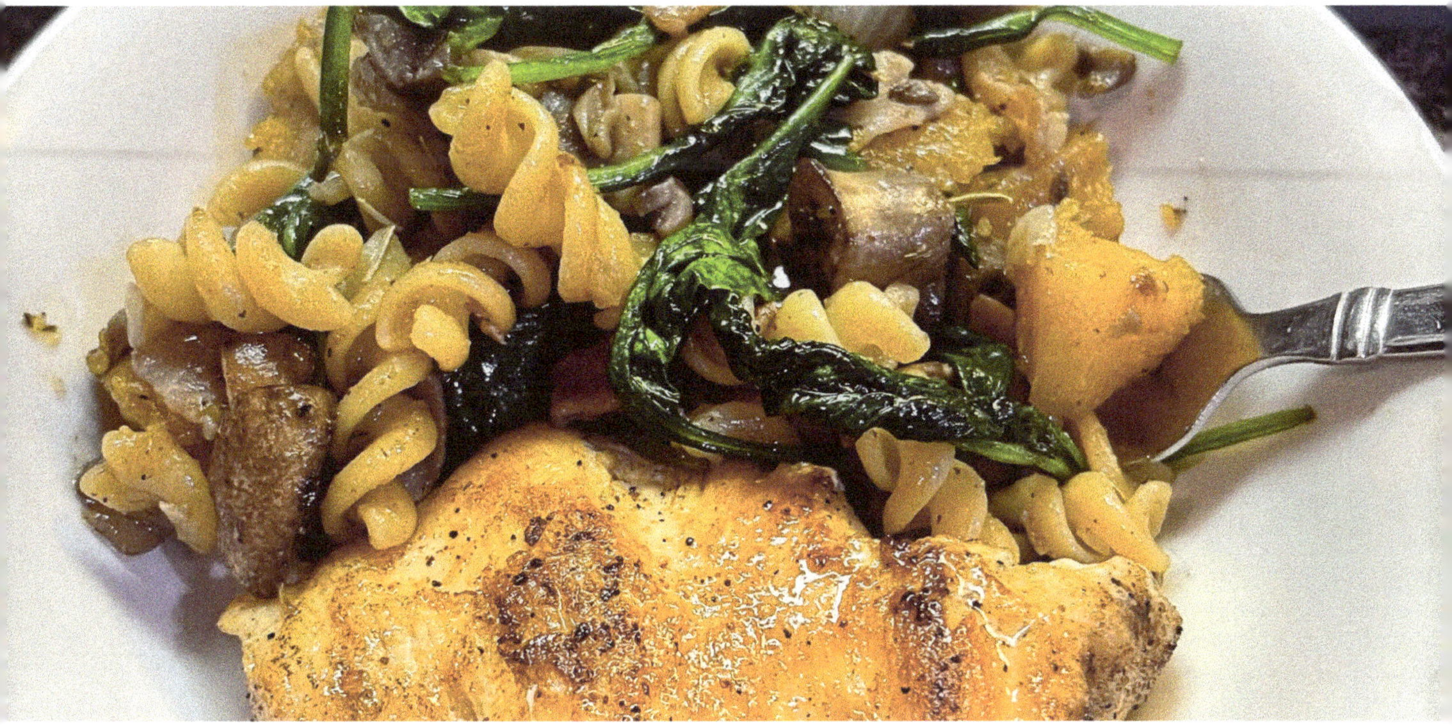

 4 servings 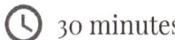 30 minutes

INGREDIENTS

- 4-6 slices uncooked bacon, chopped
- 1 lb boneless skinless chicken thighs or breasts, cut into bite-sized pieces
- ½ small onion, diced
- 2-3 cloves garlic, minced
- 1½-2 cups mushrooms, sliced
- Salt & garlic powder to taste
- 2 cups roasted butternut squash, cubed (see Dirty Side Dishes for recipe)
- 2 cups fresh spinach
- Optional: rosemary, thyme, or red pepper flakes for extra flavor
- 1 Tbsp avocado oil (optional, as needed)

DIRECTIONS

1. In a large skillet over medium heat, cook chopped bacon until crispy. Remove with a slotted spoon and set aside. Leave some rendered fat in the pan (drain excess if needed).
2. In the same skillet, add the chicken pieces. Cook until browned and cooked through, about 6-8 minutes. Remove from skillet and set aside.
3. Add the diced onions to the skillet. Sauté until softened and translucent, about 3-4 minutes.
4. Add the garlic and cook for another 30-60 seconds until fragrant.
5. Add sliced mushrooms and sauté for 6-8 minutes until browned and softened. Season with salt and garlic powder.
6. Add the roasted butternut squash cubes. Let them sit undisturbed for 2-3 minutes to get caramelized edges, then gently stir.
7. Toss in the fresh spinach and sauté until wilted, about 1-2 minutes.
8. Return the chicken and bacon to the skillet and stir to combine.
9. Optionally finish with a sprinkle of rosemary, thyme, or red pepper flakes.

This savory skillet combines roasted butternut squash, crispy bacon, earthy mushrooms, fresh spinach, and a fragrant base of sautéed garlic and onions for a rich and flavorful meal.

DAY 9
LEMON GARLIC SALMON

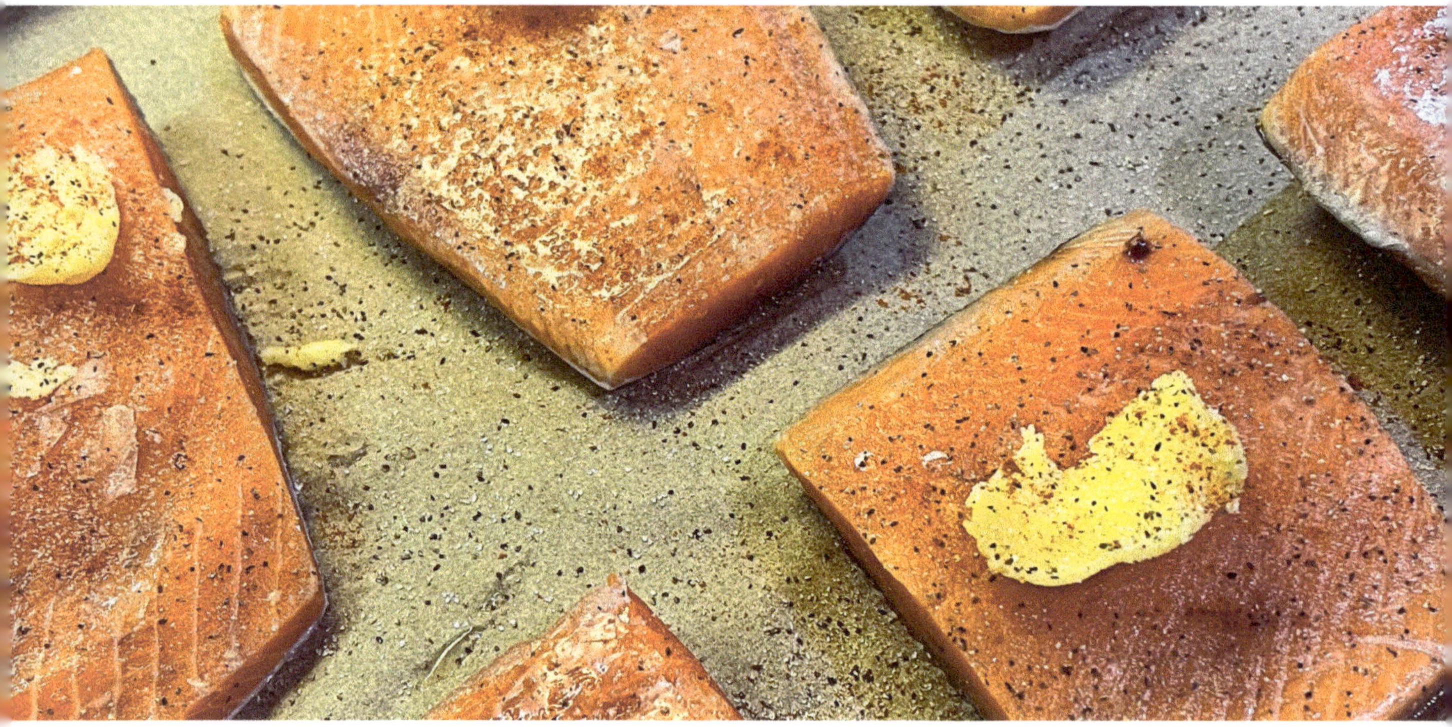

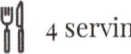 4 servings 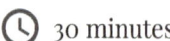 30 minutes

INGREDIENTS

- 1–2 Tbsp lemon juice
- 1 tsp lemon zest (or more to taste)
- 2 garlic cloves, minced (or 1 tsp garlic powder)
- 1 Tbsp avocado or olive oil (or ghee)
- 1 tsp dried parsley or dill (or both)
- Salt & pepper to taste
- Optional: ½ tsp coconut aminos for depth
- 1–1½ lbs salmon fillets

DIRECTIONS

1. Preheat oven to 400°F.
2. In a small bowl, mix lemon juice, lemon zest, garlic, oil, herbs, salt, pepper, and optional coconut aminos. If using ghee, omit oil and place ghee on top of fillets.
3. Rub this mixture all over the salmon fillets.
4. Place salmon in a baking dish skin down and cover loosely with foil.
5. Bake for 12–15 minutes, uncovering for the last few minutes.
6. Optional: Broil for 1–2 minutes at the end for a golden top.

Serve with The Dirty Reset™ side dishes like Sweet Potato Rounds or Cauliflower Mushroom Risotto.

DAY 10
BAKED CHICKEN WINGS

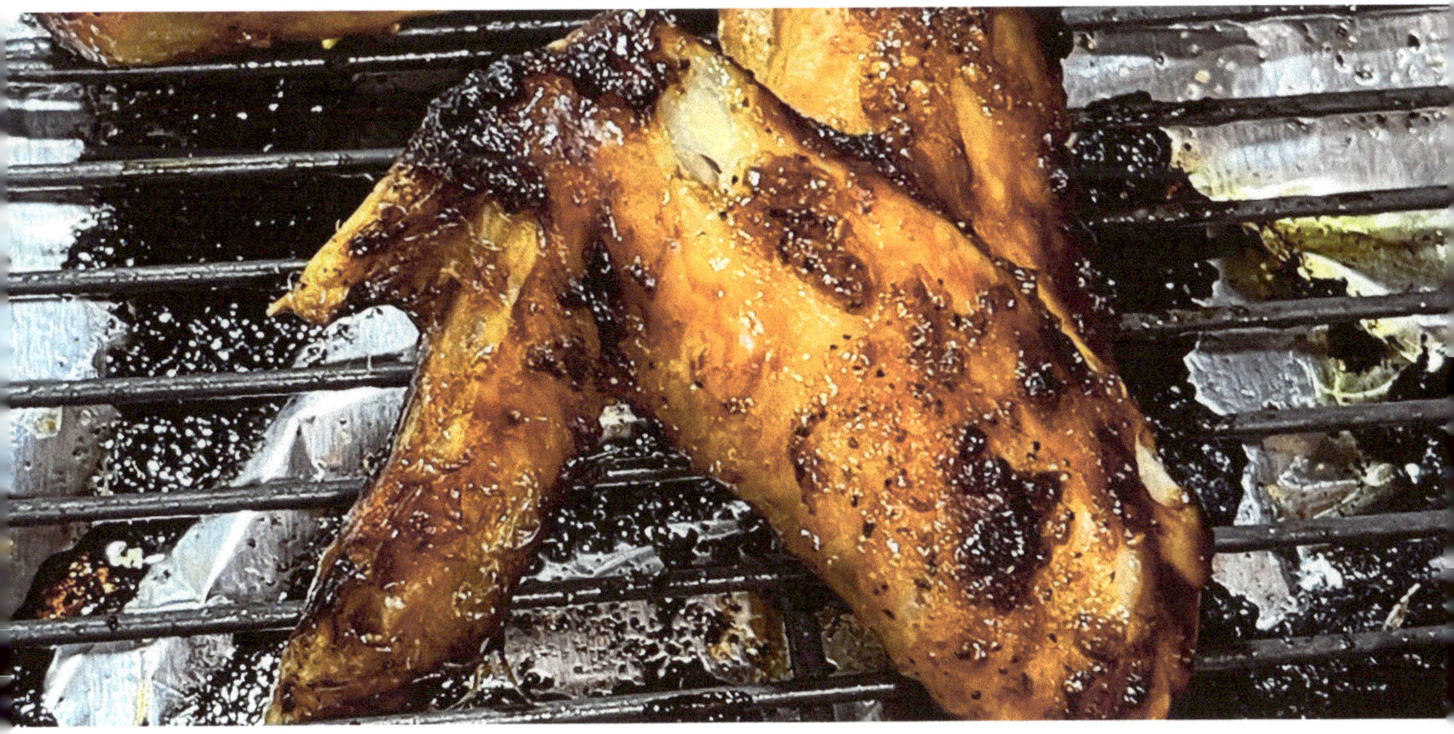

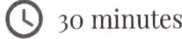 4 servings 30 minutes

INGREDIENTS

For the wings:
- 2 lbs chicken wings
- 2 Tbsp avocado or olive oil
- 1 tsp garlic powder
- 1 tsp onion powder
- 1 tsp smoked paprika
- ½ tsp salt
- ½ tsp pepper

Apricot Glaze:
- ½ cup fruit-sweetened apricot jam
- 2 Tbsp water (to thin)
- 1 tsp rice or apple cider vinegar
- ½ tsp garlic powder
- 1–2 tsp hot sauce (adjust to taste)
- Optional: pinch of cayenne pepper or crushed red pepper flakes

DIRECTIONS

1. Preheat oven to 400°F. Line a baking sheet with parchment paper or lightly grease a wire rack set over the sheet.
2. Pat chicken wings dry with paper towels.
3. In a large bowl, toss wings with oil, garlic powder, onion powder, smoked paprika, salt, and pepper.
4. In a bowl, whisk together the apricot jam, water, vinegar, garlic powder, hot sauce, and optional cayenne or red pepper flakes.
5. Generously brush glaze onto the wings you want glazed.
6. Arrange wings in a single layer on the prepared baking sheet.
7. Bake for 40–45 minutes, flipping halfway through, until wings are crispy and cooked through or until the internal temperature reaches 165°F.
8. Serve hot.

If you don't have apricot jam, you can use fruit-sweetened peach or orange marmalade instead. Perfect paired with The Dirty Reset™ Coleslaw.

DAY 11
CRAB LEGS NIGHT

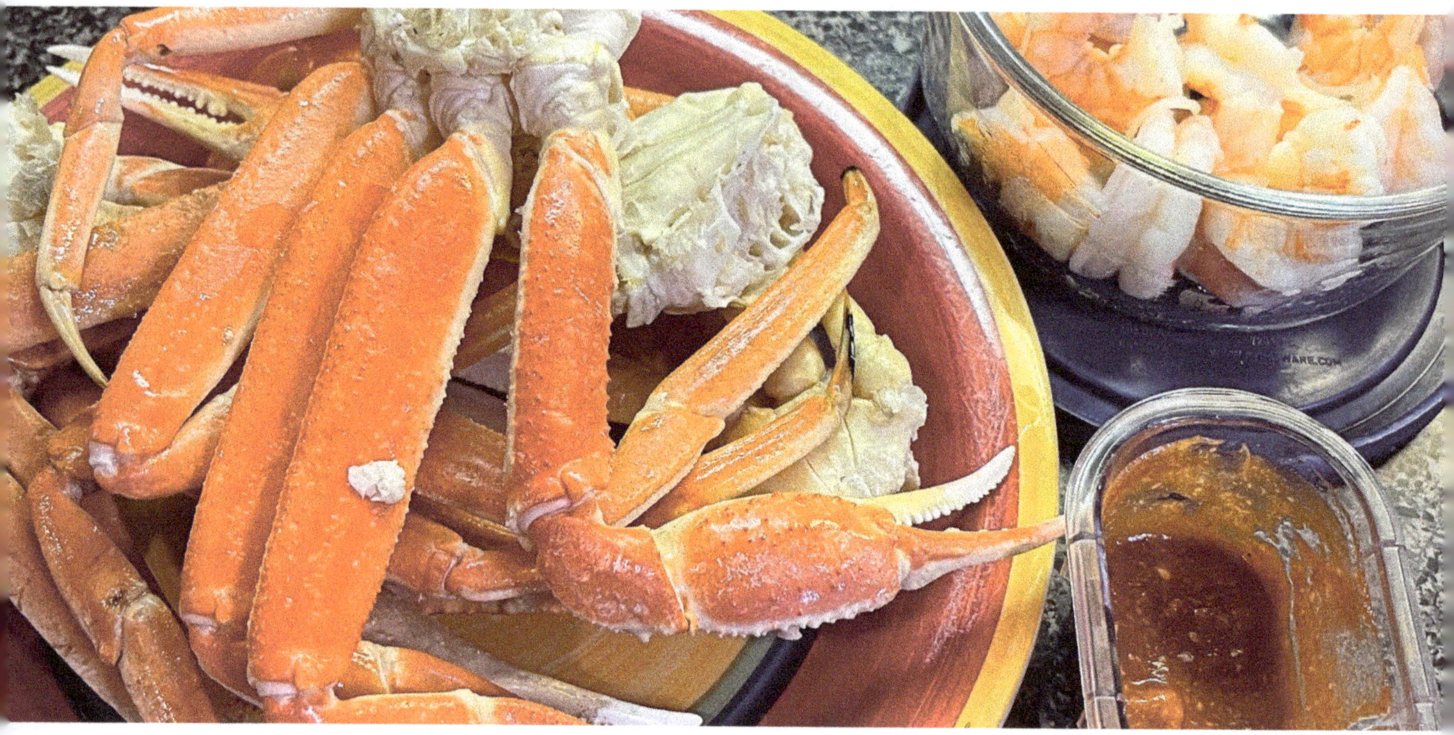

 4 servings 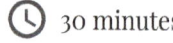 30 minutes

INGREDIENTS

For the crab legs
- Water for steaming
- 2 lbs frozen crab legs (king crab or snow crab)

For the Simple Buttery Dip
- ½ cup ghee
- 1 tsp garlic powder
- 1 tsp onion powder
- 1 tsp lemon juice
- Salt to taste
- Optional: pinch of smoked paprika or crushed red pepper flakes

DIRECTIONS

1. Fill a large stockpot with 1–2 inches of water and place a steamer basket or rack inside. Bring the water to a boil.
2. Add the frozen crab legs to the steamer basket. Cover and steam for 6–8 minutes, until heated through and fragrant. While frozen is most commonly found in stores, if using fresh/raw crab legs, steam 10–12 minutes until opaque and cooked through.
3. While the crab legs are steaming, melt ghee in a small saucepan over low heat. Stir in garlic powder, onion powder, lemon juice, and salt. Add paprika or red pepper flakes if using.
4. Remove crab legs from the pot and serve hot with Simple Buttery Dip on the side. You can also chill them and serve cold if you prefer.

> No fancy tools? Use kitchen shears or even a clean pair of scissors to cut open your crab legs.

DAY 12
STEAK & BAKED POTATOES

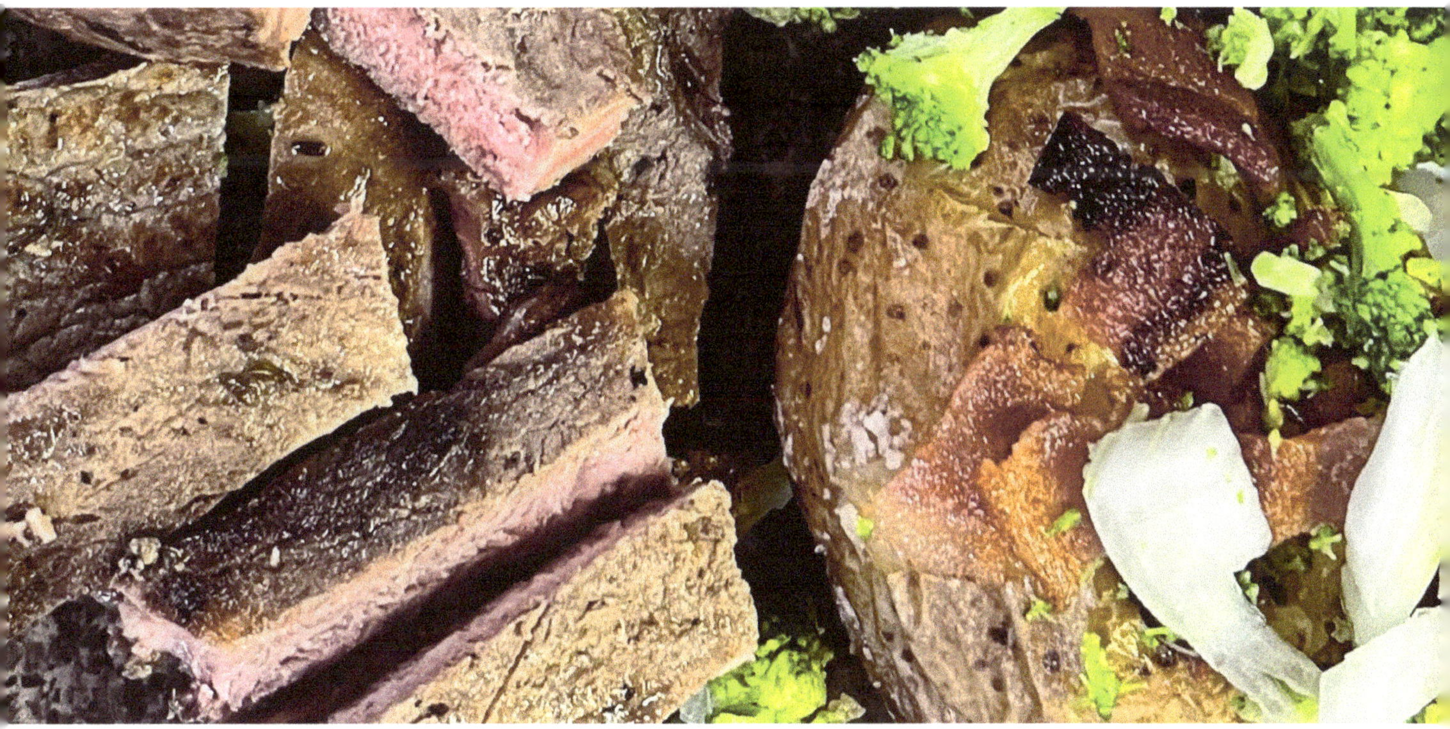

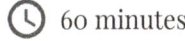

2 servings   60 minutes

INGREDIENTS

- 2 medium russet potatoes, scrubbed
- 1-2 Tbsp avocado or olive oil, divided
- Salt & pepper to taste
- Optional: garlic powder, onion powder, smoked paprika for seasoning
- 2 ribeye or strip steaks (about 8 oz each)
- Optional potato toppings: coconut aminos drizzle, chopped herbs, avocado mayo, ghee, or Cocojune yogurt

DIRECTIONS

1. Preheat oven to 400°F.
2. Lightly rub the potatoes with oil and sprinkle with salt. Pierce each several times with a fork. Place directly on the oven rack or on a baking sheet and bake for 45-60 minutes, until tender.
3. About 15 minutes before potatoes are done, season steaks generously with salt, pepper, and optional spices.
4. Heat a large cast-iron skillet over medium-high heat. Add oil.
5. Sear steaks 3-4 minutes per side for medium-rare, or to your desired doneness. Let rest 5 minutes before slicing.
6. Serve steaks with baked potatoes and your choice of optional toppings.

> Let your steak rest before slicing to keep all those tasty juices in. If your baked potato feels plain, mash it right on your plate with a drizzle of ghee or a spoonful of avocado mayo for an easy boost.

DAY 13
FRESH CHOPPED SALAD

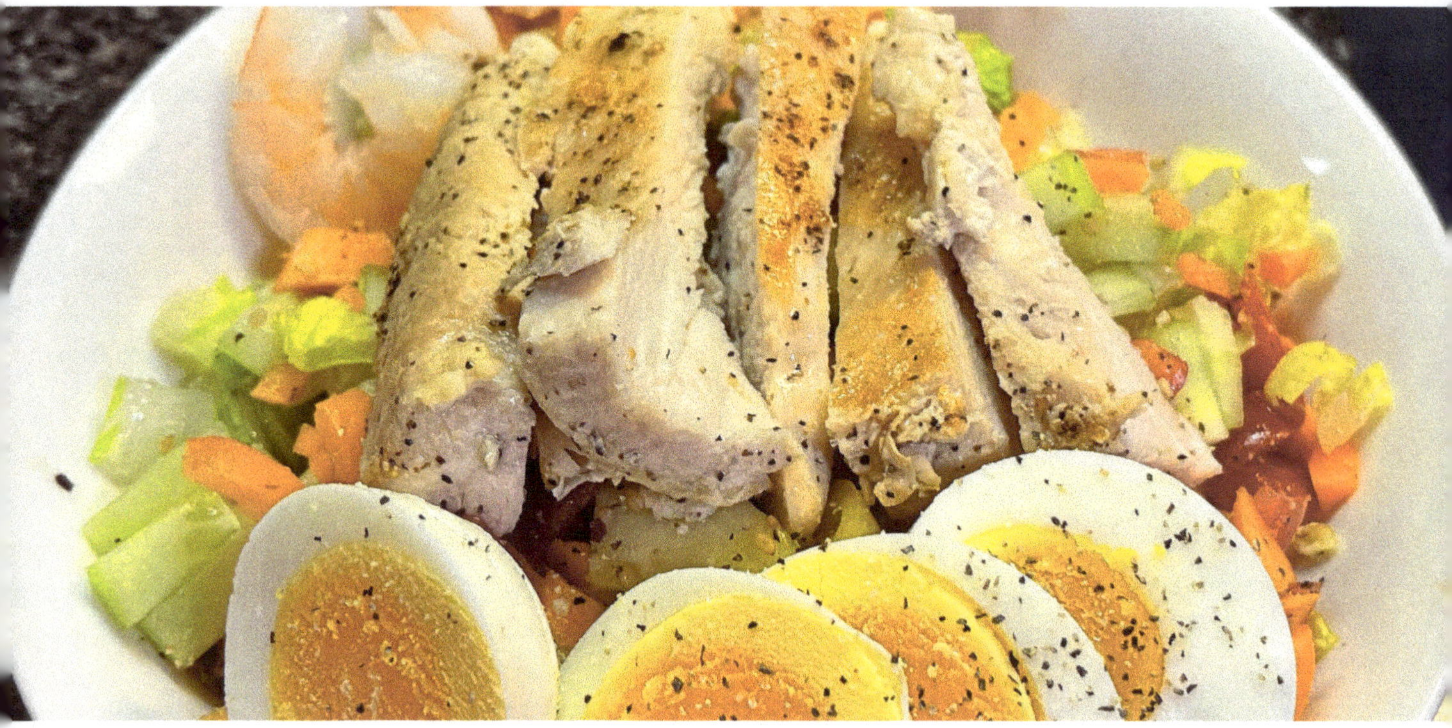

 4 servings 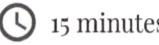 15 minutes

INGREDIENTS

- 2 cups romaine lettuce, chopped
- 1 cup cucumber, diced
- 1 cup cherry tomatoes, halved or quartered
- ½ cup bell pepper (any color), chopped
- ¼ cup red onion, finely diced (optional)
- ¼ cup carrots, chopped or shredded
- 2 Tbsp fresh herbs (parsley, dill, or basil), chopped (optional)
- Salt & pepper to taste
- The Dirty Reset™ Sweet Balsamic Salad Dressing (see The Dirty Sauce section for recipe)
- Protein option, if desired

DIRECTIONS

1. Add all vegetables to a large bowl and toss to mix.
2. Drizzle with salad dressing. Sprinkle with salt and pepper. Toss until everything is lightly coated.
3. Add in your optional protein and toss again or keep separate for serving.
4. Taste and adjust.
5. Serve immediately or chill 1 hour for flavors to meld.

Optional salad toppers:
- 1-2 hard-boiled eggs, peeled and sliced
- Grilled chicken or steak, chopped
- Shrimp, sautéed or grilled
- Canned tuna or leftover cooked salmon
- Air-fried tofu or tempeh
- 1 Tbsp chopped olives or pickles

This salad is super flexible. Mix and match based on what you have. Want crunch? Toss in chopped celery or nuts. Want creamy? Add avocado or a mayo drizzle.

DAY 14
SWEET MUSTARD MEATLOAF

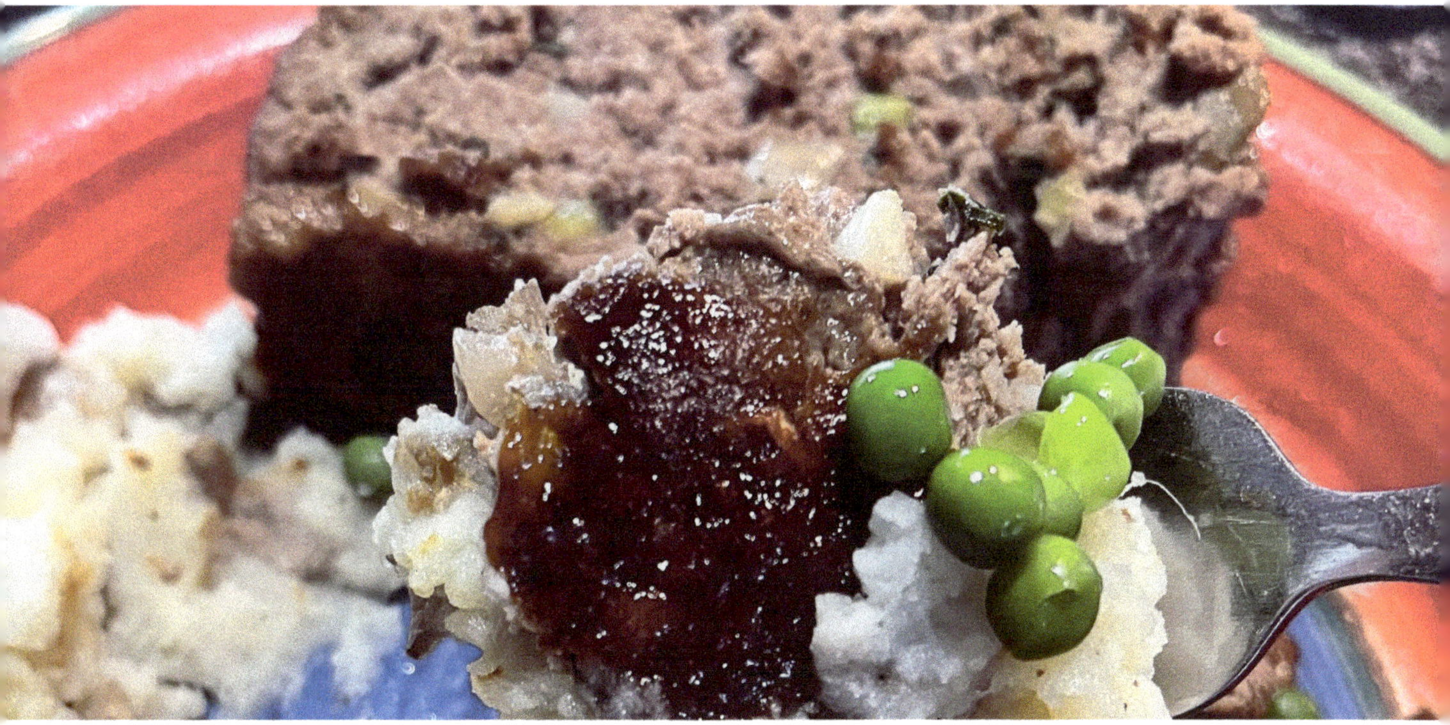

 6 servings 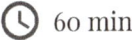 60 minutes

INGREDIENTS

Meatloaf:
- Avocado or olive oil
- ⅓ cup onion, diced
- ⅓ cup celery, diced
- ⅓ cup carrot, diced
- 2 cloves garlic, minced
- 2 lbs ground beef
- 2 eggs
- 1½ Tbsp coconut flour
- 1½ tsp coconut aminos
- 1 Tbsp mustard
- 1½ tsp poultry seasoning
- ¾ tsp salt

Mustard Glaze:
- 6 Tbsp mustard
- ¾ cup date syrup
- 2 Tbsp apple cider vinegar

DIRECTIONS

1. Preheat oven to 350°F.
2. Sauté onion, celery, carrot, and garlic in a little oil over medium heat until softened, 3–5 minutes. Let cool slightly.
3. In a large bowl, combine ground beef, eggs, sautéed vegetables, coconut flour, coconut aminos, 1 Tbsp mustard, poultry seasoning, and salt. Mix gently but don't overmix.
4. Shape into a loaf on a baking sheet or press into a loaf pan. Bake for 45 minutes.
5. Meanwhile, stir together mustard, date syrup, and apple cider vinegar for the glaze.
6. After 45 minutes, poke holes across the top of the meatloaf and spoon glaze over. Return to oven and bake 15 minutes more, or until internal temp reaches 165°F.
7. Let rest 10 minutes before slicing.

This meatloaf is packed with flavor, naturally sweetened with dates, and loaded with vegetables. It's everything you want in a comfort food dinner without the grains, dairy, or refined sugar.

DAY 15
ONE-PAN DIRTY THIGHS

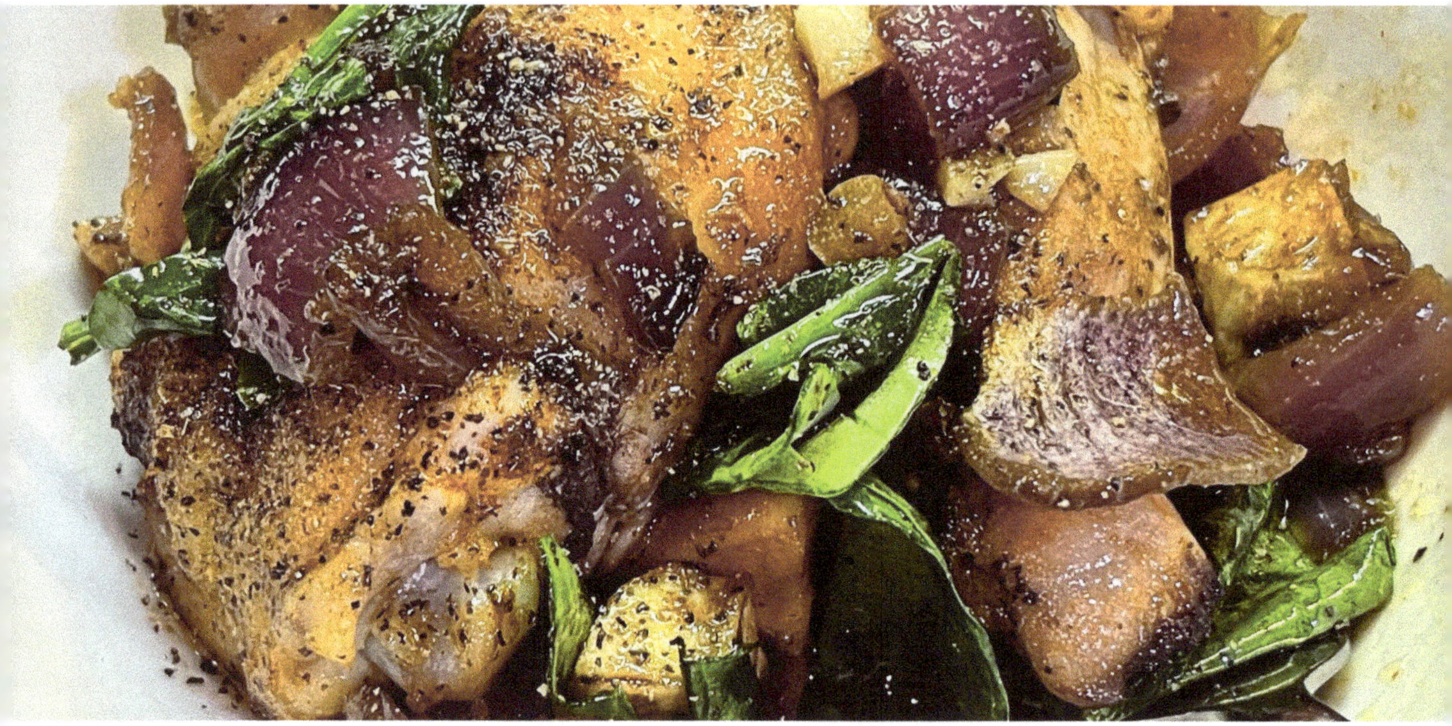

 4 servings 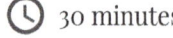 30 minutes

INGREDIENTS

- Avocado or olive oil, divided
- 1 small red onion, sliced
- 4 cloves garlic, minced
- 6 Tbsp coconut aminos
- 3 Tbsp apple cider vinegar
- 2–3 Tbsp date syrup
- 1–2 tsp garlic powder
- 6 bone-in, skin-on chicken thighs
- 2 medium sweet potatoes, diced
- 3–4 cups fresh spinach
- Salt & pepper to taste
- Optional: pinch of smoked paprika or red pepper flakes for extra flavor

DIRECTIONS

1. Preheat oven to 400°F.
2. Heat a little oil in a large oven-safe skillet over medium heat. Add the red onion and cook 2–3 minutes until starting to soften. Stir in the garlic and cook 30 seconds more, just until fragrant. Stir in coconut aminos, apple cider vinegar, date syrup, garlic powder, and a drizzle of oil. Simmer 5–7 minutes to reduce slightly.
3. Pat chicken dry and season with salt, pepper, and optional smoked paprika. Sear skin-side down in the skillet for 5–7 minutes until golden; flip and cook 2 minutes more.
4. Add sweet potatoes around the chicken and stir to coat in the sauce.
5. Transfer skillet to the oven and bake 25–30 minutes, until chicken reaches 165°F and potatoes are tender.
6. In the last 5 minutes, toss in spinach and stir to wilt.
7. Serve hot with plenty of pan sauce spooned over top.

Don't worry if the spinach looks like a lot at first — it'll cook down fast and soak up all those tasty pan juices!

DAY 16
BOLOGNESE MEAT SAUCE

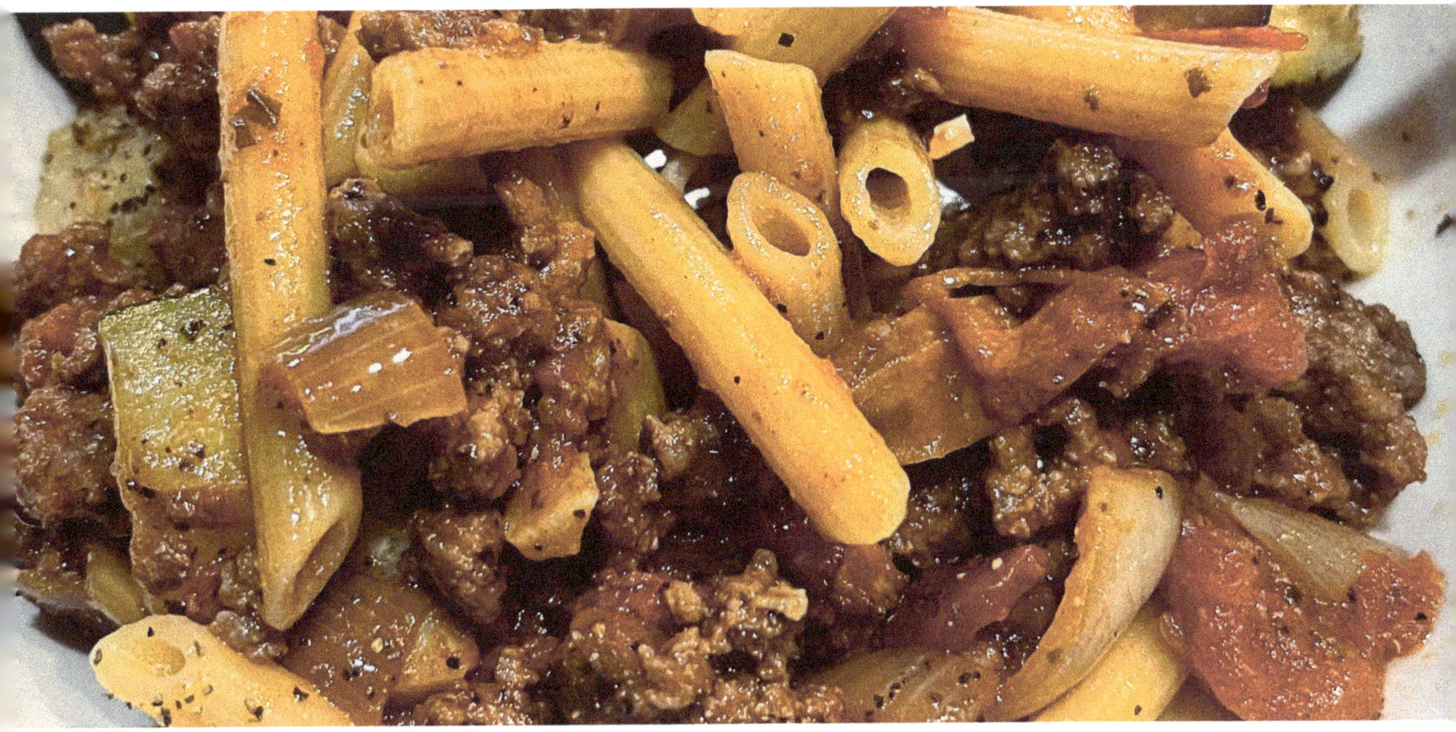

 4 servings 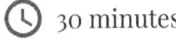 30 minutes

INGREDIENTS

- Avocado or olive oil
- 1 medium onion, diced
- 3 cloves garlic, minced
- 2 lb ground beef
- 1 can (14.5 oz) crushed tomatoes
- 1 can (14.5 oz) fire-roasted tomatoes
- 1–2 Tbsp tomato paste
- 1 Tbsp coconut aminos
- ½ to 1 tsp dried thyme
- 1 tsp dried oregano
- 1 tsp garlic powder
- 1 tsp onion powder
- Salt & pepper to taste

DIRECTIONS

1. Heat oil in a large skillet over medium heat.
2. Add diced onion and sauté until softened. Add garlic and cook for 1 more minute.
3. Add ground beef, season with salt and pepper, and cook until browned. Drain excess fat if needed.
4. Stir in crushed tomatoes, fire-roasted tomatoes, and tomato paste.
5. Add coconut aminos, dried thyme, oregano, garlic powder, and onion powder. Stir well.
6. Simmer on low heat for 20–30 minutes, stirring occasionally, until thickened to your liking.
7. Taste and adjust seasoning as needed.

> This sauce is perfect tossed with your favorite grain-free pasta or spooned over roasted veggies for an easy, hearty meal.

DAY 17
SLOW-COOKED PULLED PORK

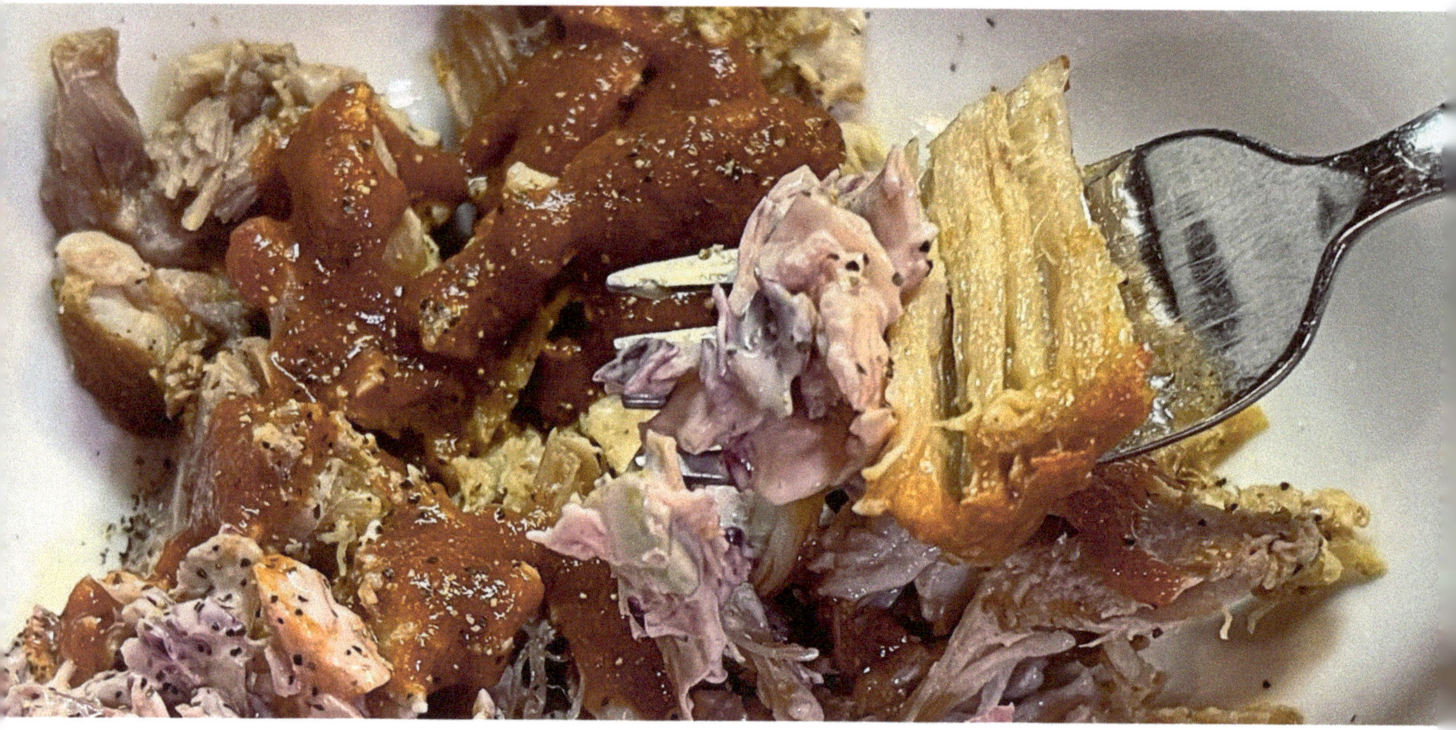

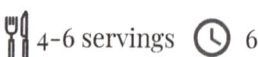

4-6 servings   6 hours

INGREDIENTS

- 1 pork roast (3 lb, shoulder or butt)
- 1 Tbsp smoked paprika
- 1½ tsp garlic powder
- 1½ tsp onion powder
- 1½ tsp salt
- 1 tsp pepper
- ½ tsp ground cumin
- ½ tsp chili powder
- ¼ tsp cayenne pepper (optional, for heat)
- ½ tsp mustard powder (optional)
- ½ Tbsp date sugar (optional, for browning at the end)
- ¼ cup broth or water (for moisture during roasting)

DIRECTIONS

1. Preheat oven to 275°F.
2. Mix all dry rub ingredients in a small bowl (excluding broth or water).
3. Pat pork roast dry with paper towels. Rub spice mix all over to coat.
4. Place in a Dutch oven or roasting pan with 1/4 cup broth or water.
5. Cover tightly with lid or foil and roast for 4 to 6 hours, until the pork is very tender and shreds easily with two forks.
6. Optional: In the last 30–45 minutes, uncover and sprinkle date sugar for browning.

This dinner goes great with The Dirty Reset™ Memphis-style BBQ sauce and Coleslaw (see The Dirty Extras sections for recipes).

DAY 18
SAUSAGE & VEGGIE SKILLET

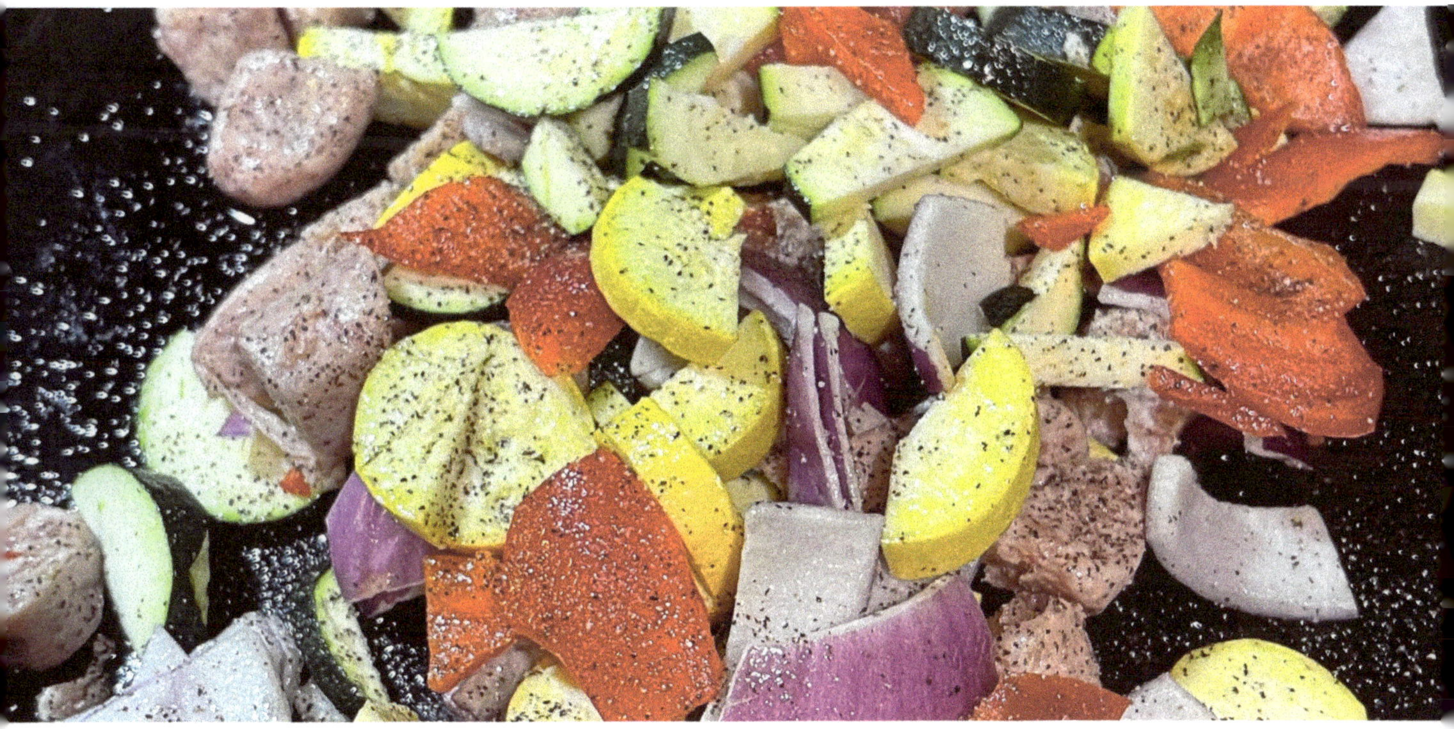

 4 servings   30 minutes

INGREDIENTS

- 1–2 Tbsp avocado or olive oil
- 4 large sausage links (no sugar added), whole or sliced into rounds
- 1 medium zucchini, diced
- 1 red bell pepper, diced
- 1 cup mushrooms, sliced
- 1 small onion, diced
- 2 cloves garlic, minced
- 2 cups fresh spinach
- Salt & pepper to taste
- Optional: pinch of red pepper flakes or smoked paprika

DIRECTIONS

1. Heat oil in a large skillet over medium heat.
2. Add sausage and cook, turning occasionally, until both sides are browned and the sausage is cooked through.
3. Add zucchini, bell pepper, and mushrooms, onion, and garlic. Sauté until vegetables are tender, about 8–10 minutes.
4. Stir in spinach and cook until wilted, about 1–2 minutes.
5. Season with salt, pepper, and optional spices. Serve hot.

This skillet is super versatile. Use whatever vegetables you have on hand. If you want to make it heartier, toss it with your favorite grain-free pasta or serve over roasted potatoes.

DAY 19
HEARTY CHILI

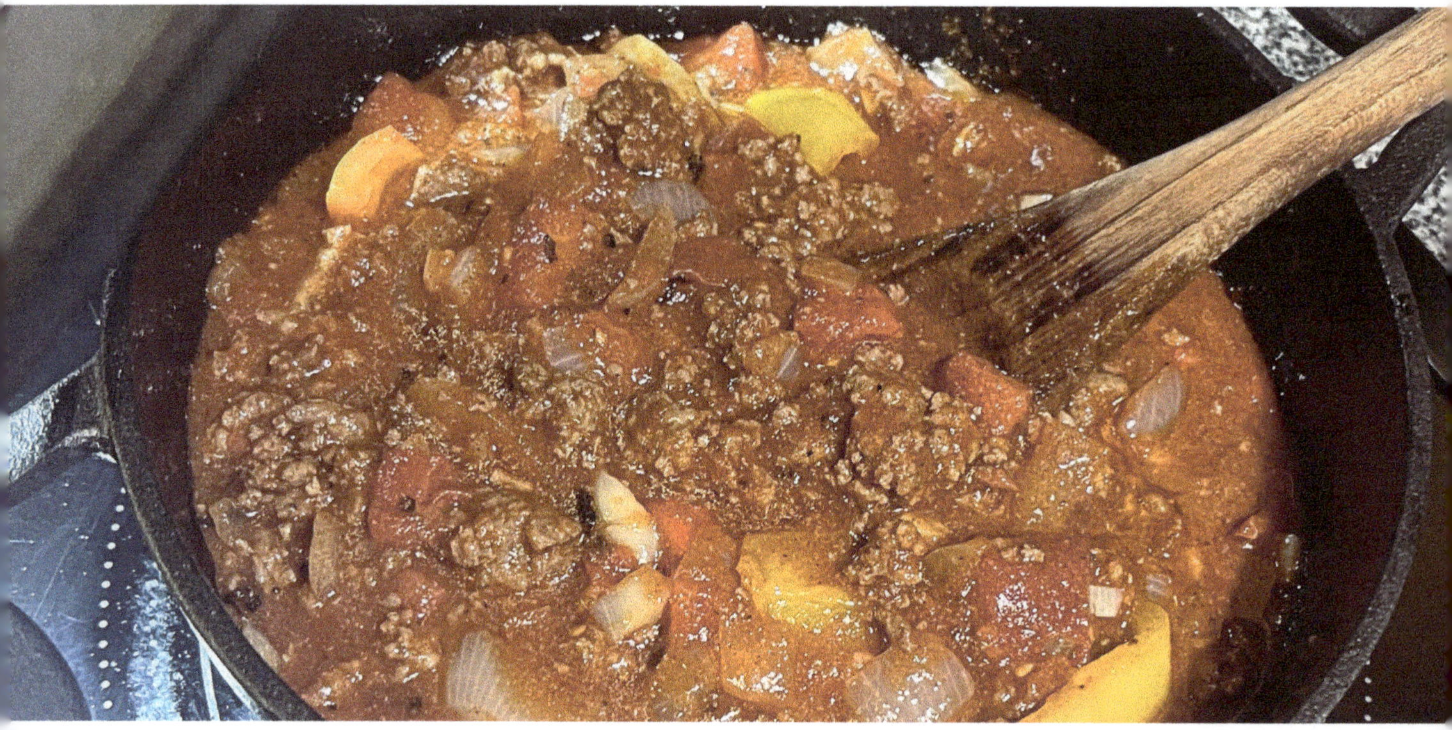

 4 servings 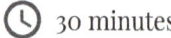 30 minutes

INGREDIENTS

- 1 lb ground beef
- Avocado or olive oil (optional, if needed)
- 1 onion, chopped
- 4 cloves garlic, minced
- 2 bell peppers, any color, chopped
- 1 can (14.5 oz) crushed tomatoes
- 1 can (14.5 oz) fire-roasted tomatoes
- 2 Tbsp tomato paste
- ½ cup beef broth or water (add more if needed)
- 1 Tbsp coconut aminos
- 1 Tbsp chili powder
- 1 tsp smoked paprika
- 1 tsp ground cumin
- ½ tsp dried oregano
- ½ tsp crushed red pepper flakes (optional, for heat)
- Salt & pepper to taste

DIRECTIONS

1. In a large pot or Dutch oven, cook the ground beef over medium heat until browned. If using lean ground beef, add a drizzle of oil first. Drain excess fat if needed; if your beef is higher in fat, you may not need extra oil.
2. Add onion, garlic, and bell peppers to the pot. Sauté for 5–7 minutes until softened.
3. Stir in tomato paste, crushed tomatoes, fire-roasted tomatoes, and beef broth. Mix well. Add coconut aminos, chili powder, smoked paprika, cumin, oregano, optional crushed red pepper flakes, salt, and pepper. Stir to combine.
4. Bring to a gentle boil, then reduce heat and simmer uncovered for 30–40 minutes, stirring occasionally, until thickened and flavorful.
5. Ladle into bowls and add your favorite toppings.

Add optional toppings like sliced green onions, diced avocado, fresh cilantro, Cocojune yogurt, or ghee drizzle.

DAY 20
KOREAN LETTUCE CUPS

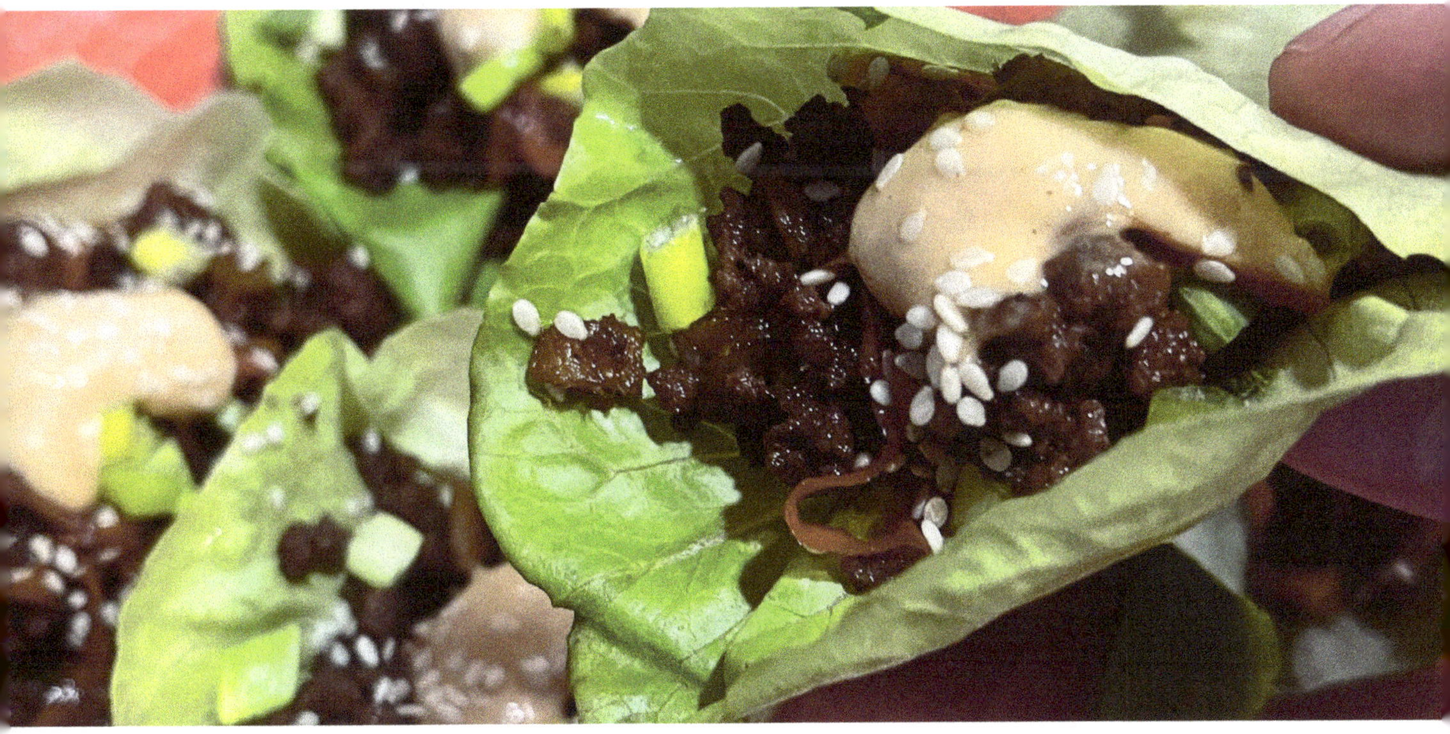

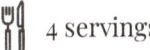 4 servings 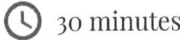 30 minutes

INGREDIENTS

- 1 lb ground beef
- 3 cloves garlic, minced
- 1 Tbsp fresh ginger, minced
- ½ cup coconut aminos
- 1–3 Tbsp date syrup
- 1 Tbsp rice vinegar
- 1 Tbsp sesame oil
- Avocado or olive oil (optional, if needed)
- Salt & pepper to taste
- Optional add-ins: ½ cup shredded carrots or 2 green onions, chopped (plus more, sliced, for garnish)
- Optional slurry: 1 tsp tapioca flour mixed with 1 Tbsp water (for a thick glossy sauce)

DIRECTIONS

1. Heat a drizzle of oil in a large skillet if using lean ground beef. Add the ground beef, garlic, and ginger. Cook over medium-high heat until the beef is browned and fully cooked, breaking it up as it cooks. Drain excess fat if needed; if your beef is higher in fat, you may not need extra oil.
2. Stir in the coconut aminos, date syrup, rice vinegar, sesame oil, and any optional vegetables such as shredded carrots or chopped green onions. Cook everything together for 5–7 minutes, stirring frequently, until the sauce thickens and coats the beef.
3. If you want a thicker, glossier sauce, slowly stir in the tapioca slurry and cook for another 1–2 minutes.
4. Serve in lettuce cups and top with sliced green onions, sesame seeds, nori strips, or pickled cucumbers, if desired.

> Nori seaweed strips, sesame seeds, and pickled veggies aren't just for looks. They add a fun crunch and pop of flavor that takes this bowl to the next level. Don't skip the toppings!

Day 21
Orange Chicken & Broccoli

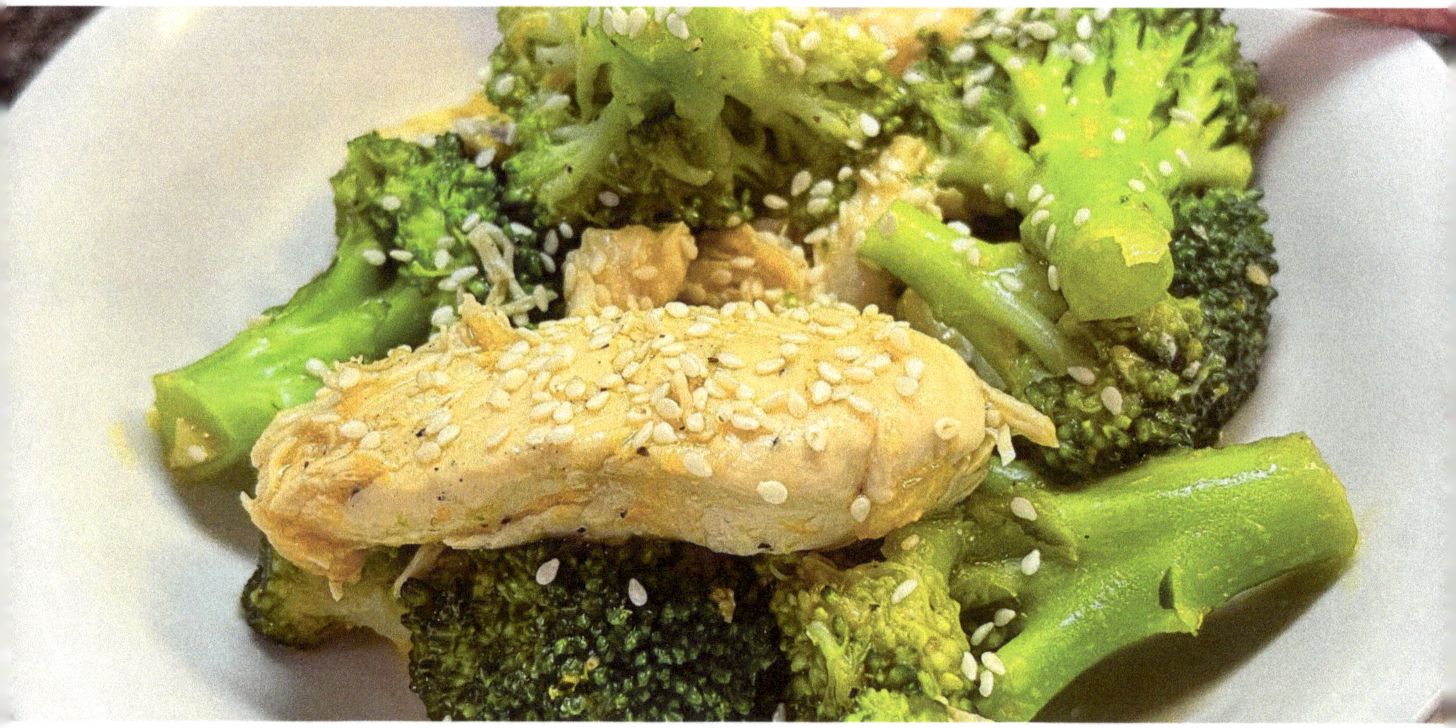

 4 servings 30 minutes

INGREDIENTS

- 1½ lbs chicken breast or tenders
- 3 cups broccoli florets
- 2-3 Tbsp avocado or olive oil, divided
- ⅓ cup orange juice
- 2 Tbsp coconut aminos
- 1 Tbsp apple cider vinegar
- 1 tsp garlic powder
- ½ tsp ground ginger
- ½ tsp salt (or to taste)
- ¼ tsp pepper
- Optional: 1 tsp tapioca flour mixed with 1 Tbsp water (for thickening)

DIRECTIONS

1. Heat 1-2 Tbsp oil in a large skillet over medium-high heat. Add the chicken and cook until browned and cooked through. Remove from the skillet and set aside.
2. Add the remaining oil to the skillet if needed. Toss in the broccoli and stir-fry for 3-4 minutes until bright green and just crisp-tender.
3. In a small bowl, whisk together the orange juice, coconut aminos, apple cider vinegar, garlic powder, ginger, salt, and pepper.
4. Return the chicken to the skillet and pour the sauce over the chicken and broccoli. Cook for 1-2 minutes, stirring gently, until everything is coated.
5. If you want a thicker sauce, whisk the tapioca flour with water in a small bowl to make a slurry. Slowly stir it into the skillet and cook for another 1-2 minutes until the sauce thickens slightly.
6. Serve hot.

Stir-fry the broccoli briefly at high heat, which keeps it bright green with a nice crisp bite so it won't get mushy.

DAY 22
FISH CHOWDER

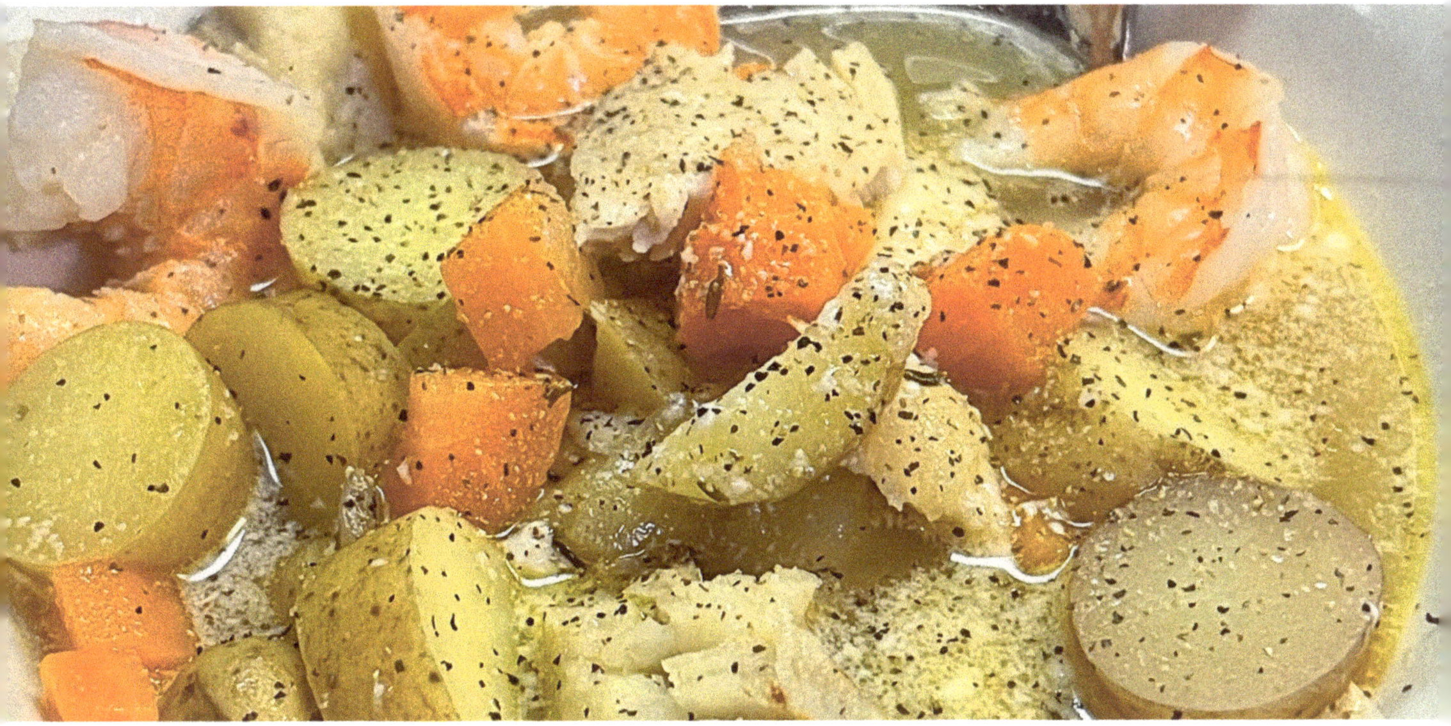

 4 servings 30 minutes

INGREDIENTS

- 1–2 Tbsp avocado oil or ghee
- 1 medium onion, diced
- 2 cloves garlic, minced
- 2–3 stalks celery, diced
- 1 cup carrots, diced
- 3 medium potatoes, diced
- ½ tsp dried thyme
- ½ tsp smoked paprika
- Salt & pepper to taste
- 4 cups chicken broth
- 1 can (13.5 oz) full-fat coconut milk
- 1 lb white fish fillets (fresh or frozen)
- Optional: bay leaf
- Optional: peeled shrimp
- Optional: fresh parsley

DIRECTIONS

1. Heat avocado oil or ghee in a large pot over medium heat. Add onions, garlic, celery, and carrots. Sauté for 5–7 minutes, until softened.
2. Add potatoes, thyme, smoked paprika, and a good pinch of salt and pepper. Stir well to coat.
3. Pour in chicken broth and bring to a boil. Reduce heat and simmer for 10–15 minutes, until potatoes are tender.
4. Stir in the coconut milk and add the fish fillets. If using frozen fillets, add them directly to the pot and cook until opaque and flaky. After the fish has simmered for 3–4 minutes, add the optional peeled shrimp and continue cooking 2–3 minutes more, until the shrimp are pink and opaque.
5. Simmer gently for 5–7 minutes, until the fish is cooked through.
6. Taste and adjust seasoning as needed.
7. Remove bay leaf if used. Serve hot, garnished with fresh parsley if desired.

Don't stress about peeling the potatoes. The skin adds a little texture and extra nutrients. Frozen fish works just fine, and there's no need to thaw.

DAY 23
EGG ROLL BOWL

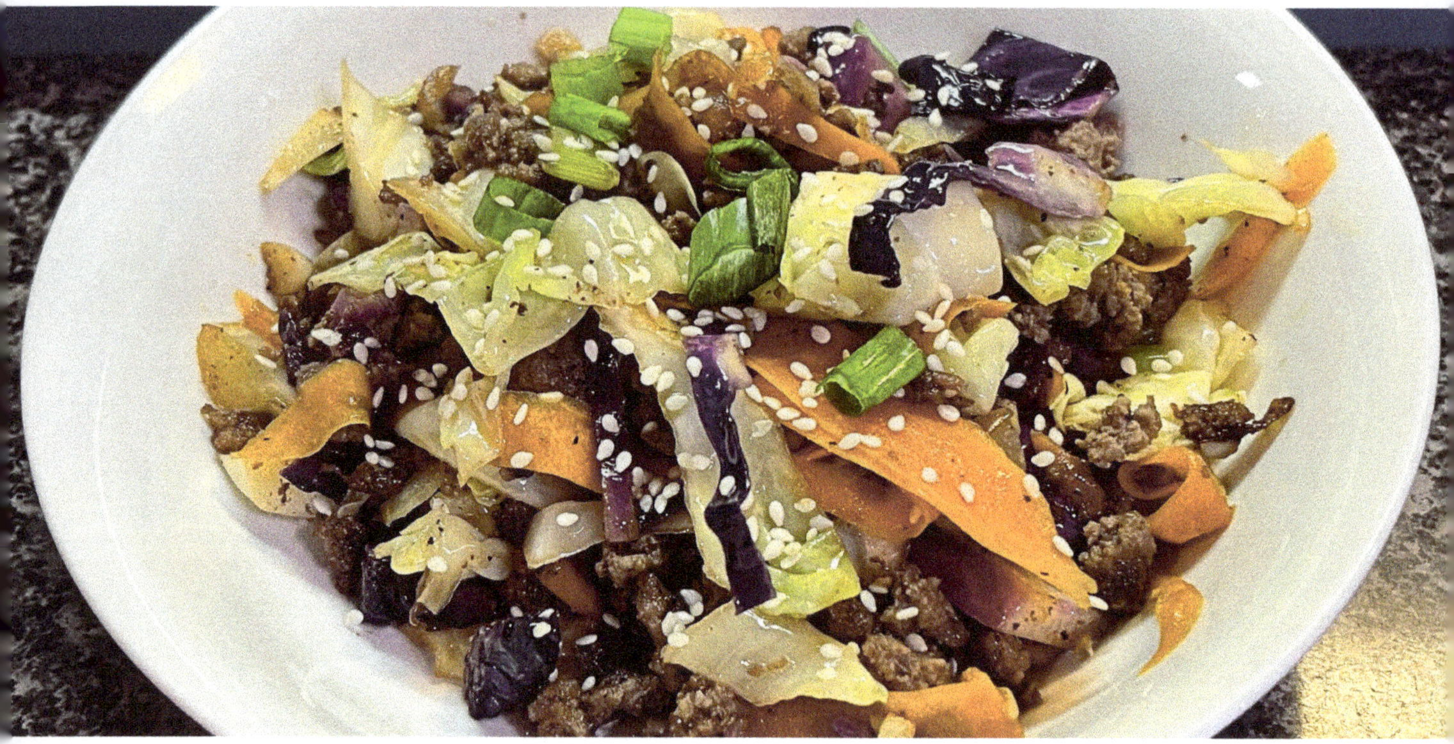

 4 servings 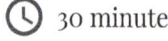 30 minutes

INGREDIENTS

- Avocado or olive oil (for cooking)
- 1 lb shrimp or thinly sliced chicken breast
- 1 small onion, thinly sliced
- 3 cloves garlic, minced
- 1 Tbsp fresh ginger, minced
- 1 bell pepper, thinly sliced
- 2 cups cabbage, shredded
- 1 large carrot, julienned
- 2 cups zucchini or sweet potato, diced or spiralized
- 3 Tbsp coconut aminos
- 1 Tbsp rice vinegar
- 1 Tbsp lime juice
- 1 Tbsp sesame oil
- Salt & pepper to taste
- Optional toppings: fresh cilantro, lime wedges, sliced green onions, sesame seeds, chopped cashews, sriracha

DIRECTIONS

1. Heat a drizzle of oil in a large skillet over medium-high heat.
2. Add the shrimp or chicken along with the onion, garlic, ginger, and bell pepper. Cook 4–5 minutes, stirring frequently, until the shrimp turns pink (or the chicken is mostly cooked through) and the vegetables begin to soften.
3. Add the shredded cabbage, carrot, and zucchini noodles or sweet potatoes. Stir in the coconut aminos, rice vinegar, lime juice, sesame oil, salt, and pepper.
4. Continue cooking 5–7 minutes more, tossing occasionally, until the vegetables are tender-crisp and the shrimp or chicken is fully cooked.
5. Serve hot, topped with fresh cilantro, lime wedges, sliced green onions, sesame seeds, chopped cashews, or a drizzle of sriracha if desired.

For an extra boost of flavor, try topping this bowl with a drizzle of The Dirty Reset™ Yum Yum Fusion Sauce. See The Dirty Sauce section for recipe.

DAY 24
CHICKEN SOUP

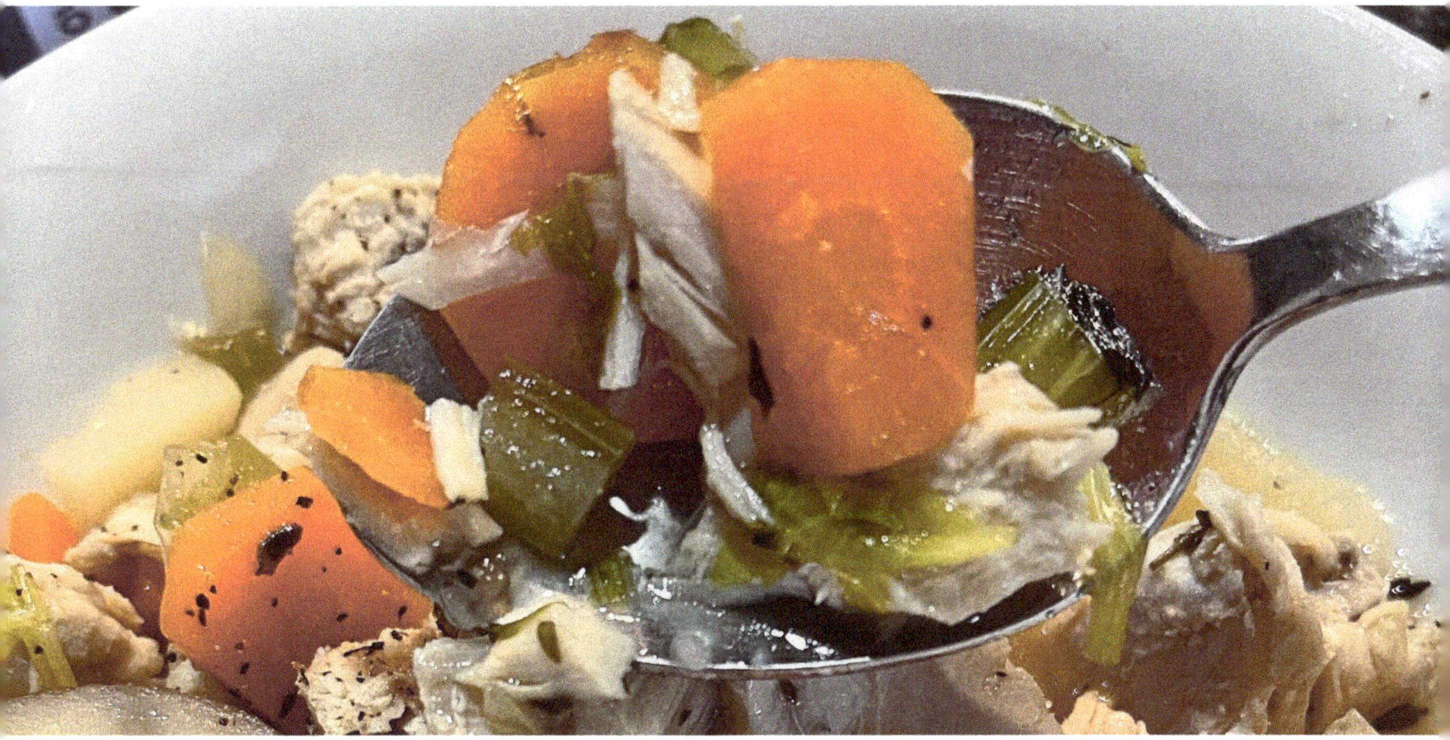

 4 servings 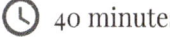 40 minutes

INGREDIENTS

- 1–2 Tbsp avocado or olive oil (for sautéing)
- 1 medium onion, diced
- 2–3 cloves garlic, minced
- 3 ribs celery, diced
- 3 medium carrots, peeled & sliced
- 2 medium potatoes, peeled & diced
- 8 cups chicken broth
- 1 tsp dried thyme (or Italian seasoning)
- 1 bay leaf (optional)
- Salt & pepper to taste
- 2 large cooked chicken breasts, shredded or chopped (try using your Oven-Baked Chicken recipe from Day 3)

DIRECTIONS

1. In a large pot, heat oil over medium heat. Add the onion and garlic; cook for 3-4 minutes until softened and fragrant.
2. Add the celery and carrots and cook 3-4 minutes more, stirring occasionally.
3. Pour in the chicken broth, add the potatoes, thyme, bay leaf, salt, and pepper. Bring to a boil.
4. Reduce to a simmer and cook for 20-25 minutes, until the potatoes and carrots are fork-tender.
5. Stir in the cooked chicken and simmer another 5-10 minutes to heat through.
6. Remove the bay leaf, taste, and adjust seasoning as needed.

> This soup is perfect for freezing, so save some for a rainy day.
> A splash of lemon, a dash of hot sauce, or a sprinkle of parsley makes it feel extra warm and fresh.

Day 25
CIDER-KISSED PORK CHOPS

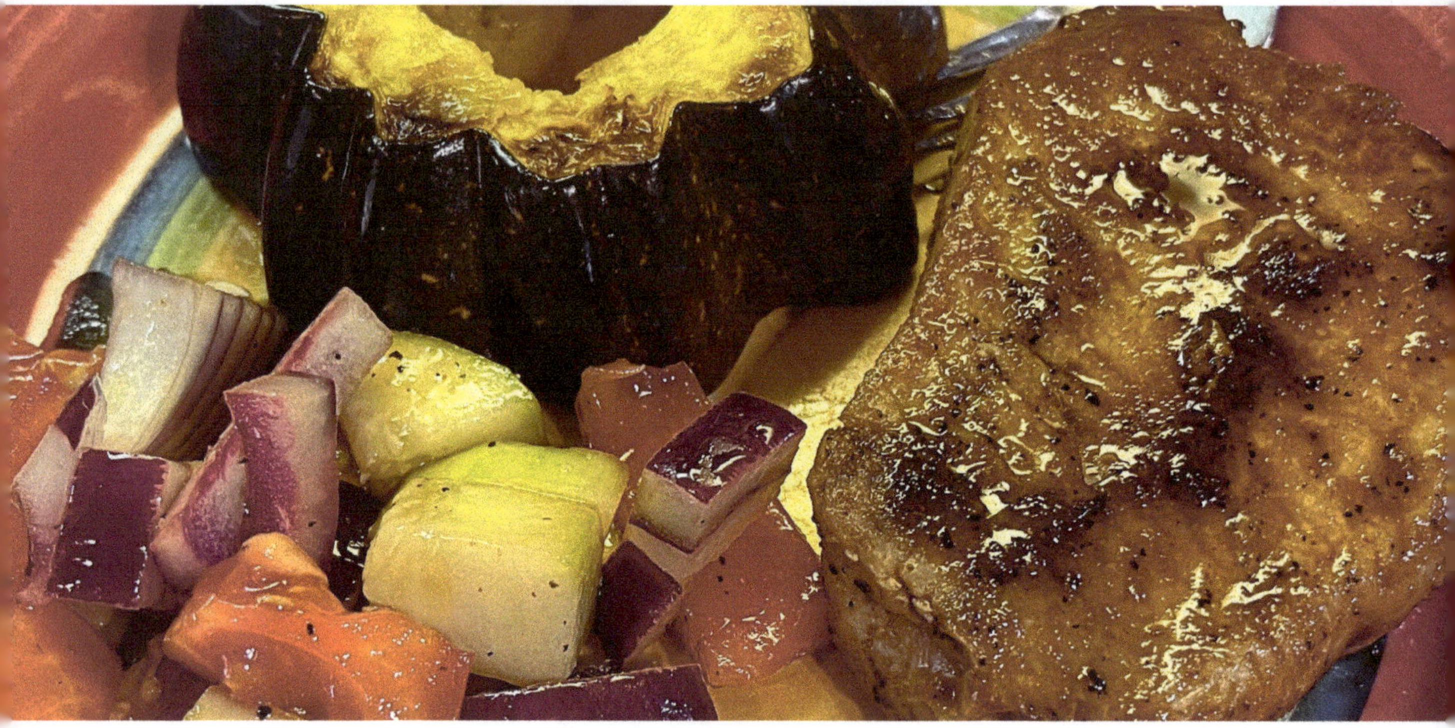

 4 servings 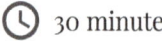 30 minutes

INGREDIENTS

- 3–4 pork chops (bone-in or boneless, about 1 inch thick)
- 2 Tbsp avocado or olive oil
- 1 tsp salt
- 1 tsp garlic powder (for seasoning rub)
- ½ tsp pepper
- 1 tsp smoked paprika
- ½ cup apple cider vinegar
- 3 Tbsp coconut aminos
- 1–2 Tbsp date syrup (optional, for sweetness)
- 2 cloves garlic, minced (or 1 tsp garlic powder, for glaze)

DIRECTIONS

1. Pat pork chops dry and season both sides with salt, garlic powder, pepper, and smoked paprika.
2. Heat oil in a skillet over medium-high heat. Sear the pork chops for 3–4 minutes per side, working in batches if needed, until golden brown.
3. Remove chops and set aside (they'll finish cooking in the glaze).
4. In the same skillet, add apple cider vinegar, coconut aminos, date syrup, and minced garlic.
5. Simmer for 2–3 minutes until the glaze starts to reduce.
6. Return pork chops to the skillet and cook for another 4–6 minutes, spooning glaze over the top, until cooked through (145°F internal temp).
7. Let rest 5 minutes before serving. Spoon extra glaze over the top.

A tangy-sweet twist on classic pork chops.
This glaze uses apple cider vinegar and coconut aminos for a bold flavor.

DAY 26
SEAFOOD NIGHT

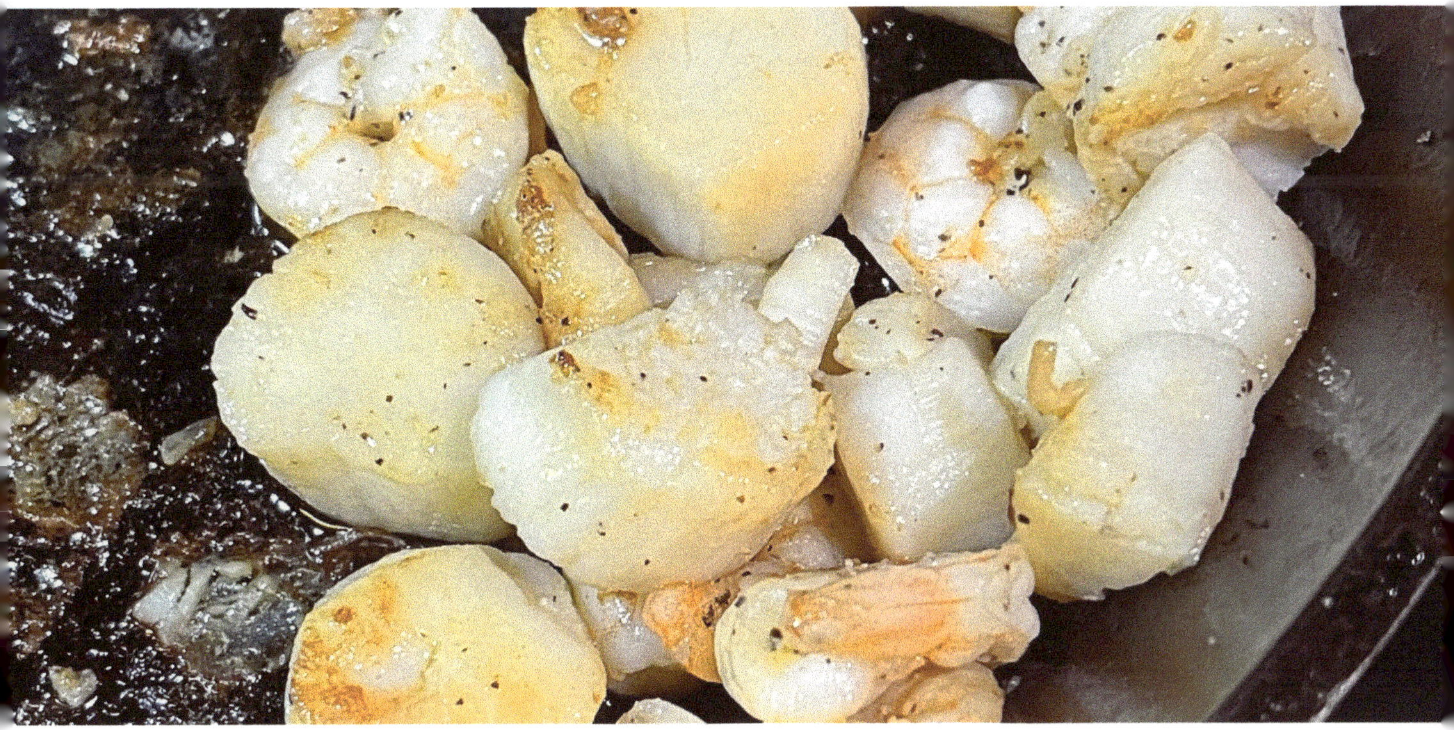

 4 servings 30 minutes

INGREDIENTS

- 2–3 Tbsp avocado or olive oil
- ½ lb shrimp, peeled & deveined
- ½ lb scallops
- ½ lb firm white fish, cut into chunks
- 2 cloves garlic, minced
- 2 Tbsp lemon juice
- 2 Tbsp coconut aminos
- ½ tsp smoked paprika
- ½ tsp salt (or to taste)
- ¼ tsp pepper
- Optional: pinch of red pepper flakes, fresh herbs

DIRECTIONS

1. Heat oil in a large skillet over medium-high heat.
2. Add shrimp, scallops, and fish in a single layer. Season with salt, pepper, smoked paprika, and garlic.
3. Cook 2–3 minutes without stirring so you get a nice sear.
4. Gently toss or turn the seafood. Add lemon juice and coconut aminos.
5. Continue cooking another 4–5 minutes, until shrimp are pink, scallops are opaque, and fish flakes easily.
6. Serve hot, spooning pan juices over the seafood.

Serve this with roasted vegetables or your favorite side dishes. Just be careful not to overcook the seafood so it stays juicy and tender.

DAY 27
CURRY & MASHED POTATOES

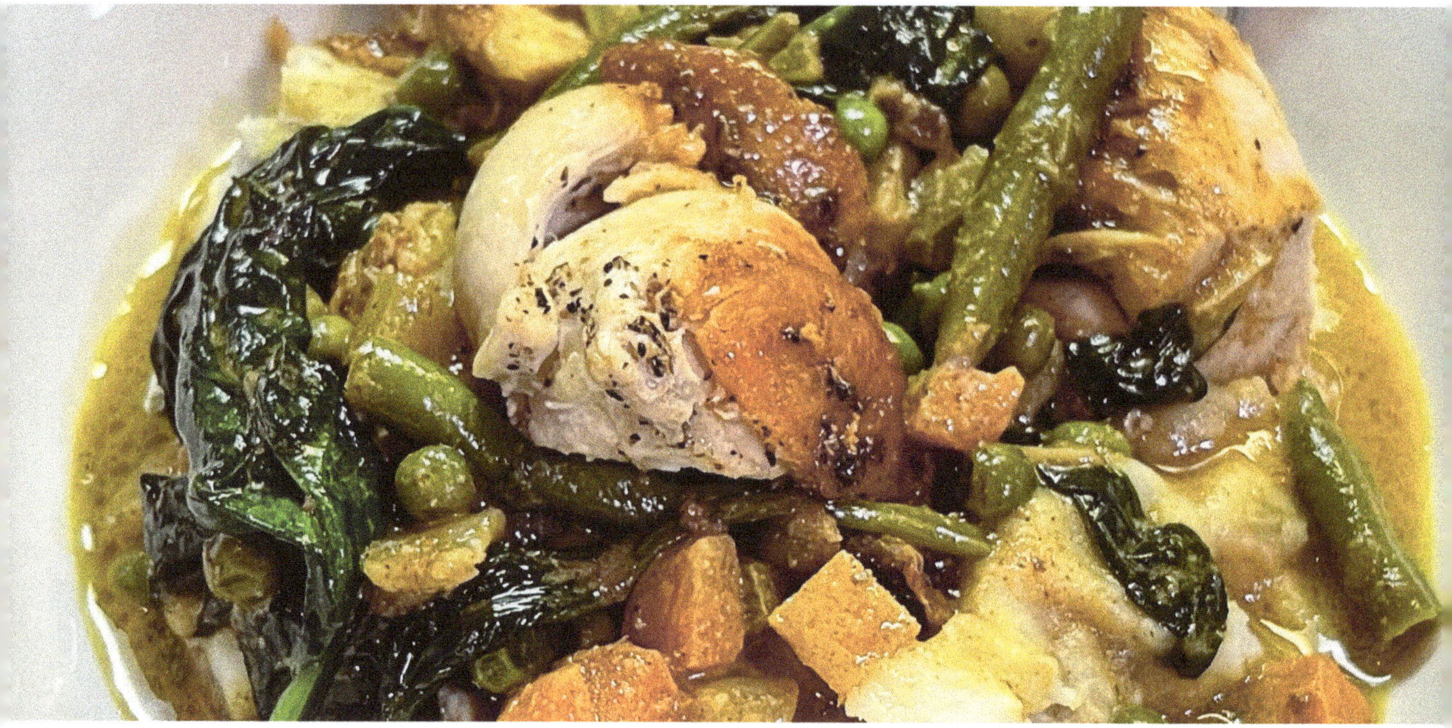

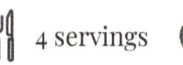 4 servings 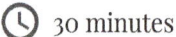 30 minutes

INGREDIENTS

- 2–3 Tbsp avocado or olive oil
- 1½ lbs chicken or lamb (cut into bite-size pieces)
- 1 can (13.5 oz) full-fat coconut milk
- 2 cups mixed vegetables (fresh or frozen)
- 2–3 cups fresh spinach

Spice Mix:
- 2 tsp curry powder
- 1 tsp cumin
- ½ tsp allspice
- ¼ tsp ground cloves
- ½ tsp cinnamon
- 1 tsp salt (or to taste)
- ½ tsp pepper
- 1 tsp garlic powder
- ½ tsp paprika
- ¼ tsp nutmeg
- ½ tsp turmeric
- ½ tsp ground mustard
- Optional: red pepper flakes or cayenne for heat

DIRECTIONS

1. Heat oil in a large skillet over medium-high heat. Add chicken or lamb and cook until browned and cooked through.
2. In a bowl, whisk together coconut milk with curry powder, cumin, allspice, cloves, cinnamon, salt, pepper, garlic powder, paprika, nutmeg, turmeric, and mustard.
3. Add frozen mixed vegetables to the skillet with the cooked meat.
4. Pour the spiced coconut milk mixture over the meat and vegetables in the skillet. Stir to combine.
5. Bring to a gentle simmer and cook until the sauce starts to thicken, about 7–10 minutes.
6. Stir in fresh spinach and cook until wilted (about 1–2 minutes).
7. Serve hot, spooning extra sauce over the top.

> Swap in any vegetables you have on hand and try it over The Dirty Reset™ mashed potatoes to soak up that delicious sauce (see the Dirty Side Dishes section for recipe).

DAY 28
SLOW-BAKED RIBS

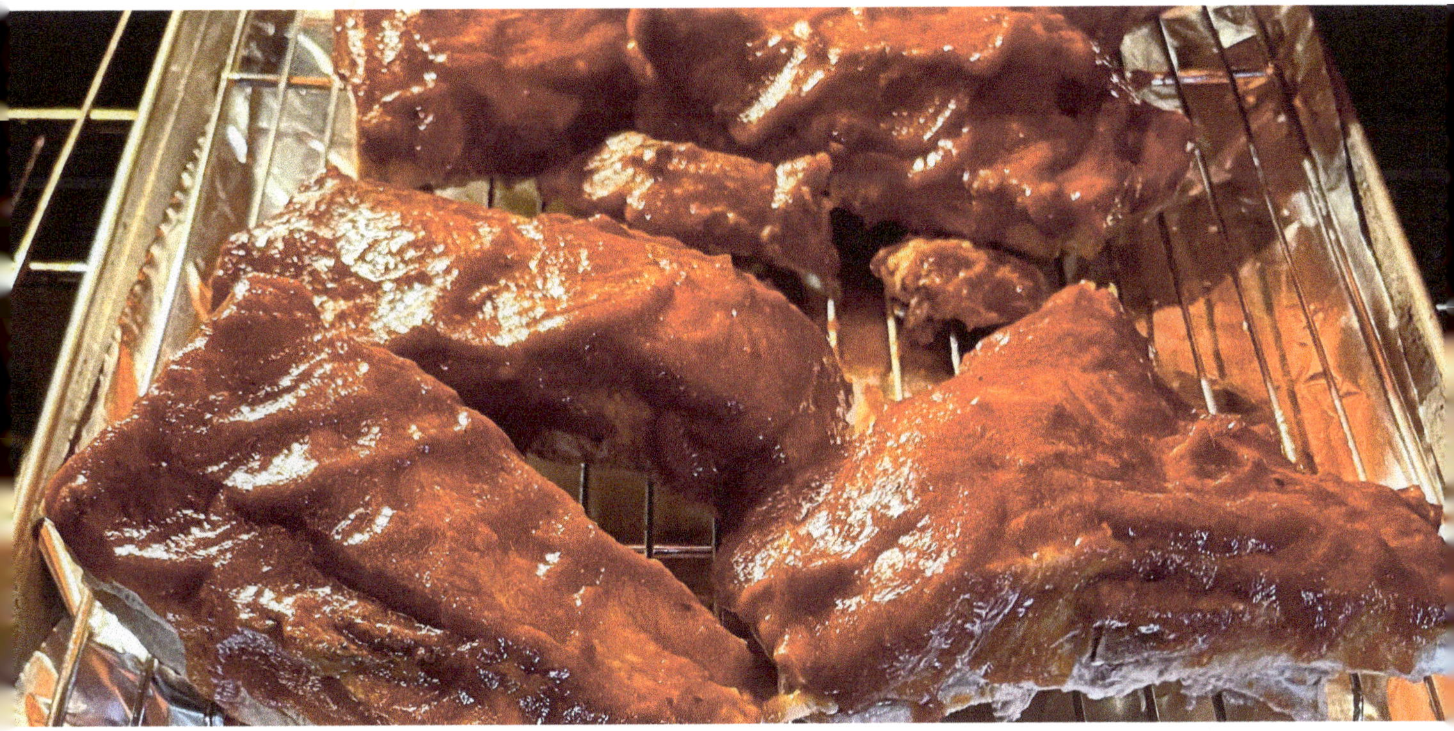

 6 servings 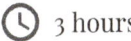 3 hours

INGREDIENTS

- 1 rack pork ribs (about 2–3 lbs)
- Salt & pepper to taste
- Optional: ½–1 tsp each garlic powder, smoked paprika, and onion powder
- The Dirty Reset™ BBQ Sauce (see The Dirty Sauce section for recipe)

DIRECTIONS

1. Preheat oven to 300°F. Line a baking sheet with foil.
2. Pat the ribs dry with paper towels. Season both sides generously with salt, pepper, and any optional seasonings you like. Place on the prepared baking sheet, cover tightly with foil, and bake for 2½ to 3 hours, until tender.
3. After baking, brush ribs generously with The Dirty Reset BBQ Sauce.
4. Broil or bake at 425°F for 10–15 minutes, until caramelized.
5. Slice between the bones and serve hot.

For extra flavor, brush on a second layer of sauce halfway through caramelizing. It gives the ribs a sticky, finger-licking glaze!

DAY 29
SWEET & SPICY MANGO SHRIMP

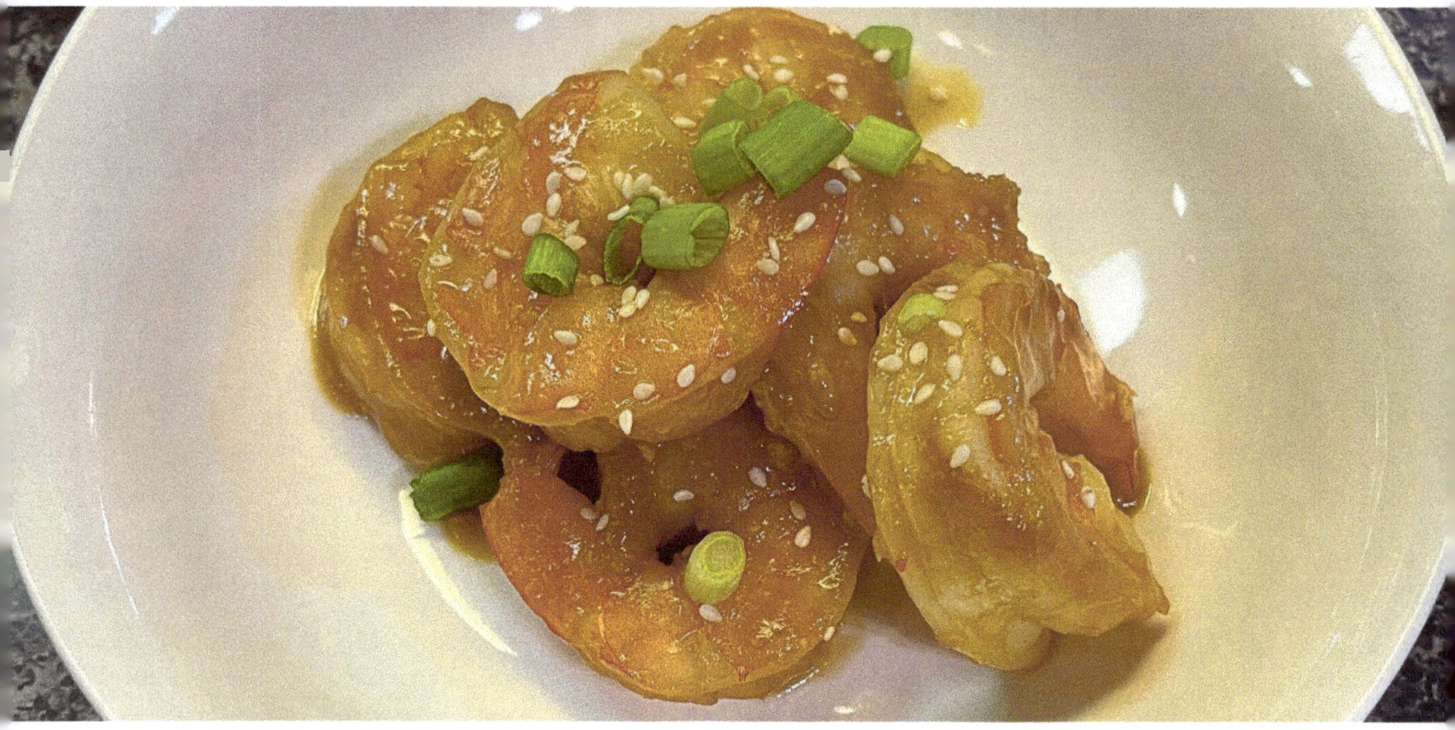

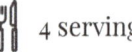 4 servings 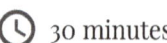 30 minutes

INGREDIENTS

- 1 Tbsp avocado or olive oil
- 1 lb raw shrimp, peeled & deveined (tail-on optional)
- ½ cup mango purée (from 1 small ripe mango, mashed, or from thawed and blended frozen mango chunks)
- 2 Tbsp coconut aminos
- 1 Tbsp apple cider vinegar
- 1–2 tsp hot sauce or ⅛ tsp cayenne pepper
- 3 cloves garlic, minced
- ½ tsp fresh ginger, grated (or ¼ tsp ground ginger)
- Pinch of salt, to taste
- Juice of ½ lime (optional, for extra brightness)
- Optional garnish: sliced green onions & sesame seeds

DIRECTIONS

1. Peel and devein shrimp before cooking. Keep tails on if you like the look, but remove all shells so sauce will fully coat the meat. Pat shrimp dry with paper towels.
2. In a bowl, whisk together the mango purée, coconut aminos, vinegar, hot sauce or cayenne, garlic, ginger, and lime juice (if using). Set aside.
3. Heat oil in a large skillet over medium-high heat. Add shrimp in a single layer and cook for 2–3 minutes per side until just pink and opaque.
4. Reduce heat to medium. Pour sauce into the skillet and toss to coat. Simmer for 2–3 minutes until the sauce thickens slightly.
5. Taste and adjust seasoning. Garnish with green onions and sesame seeds.

No mango? Try blended peach or pineapple for a tasty twist. You can also use no-sugar-added mango baby food or a packaged mango sauce, like Golden Farms Organic Mango Sauce, as a quick shortcut.

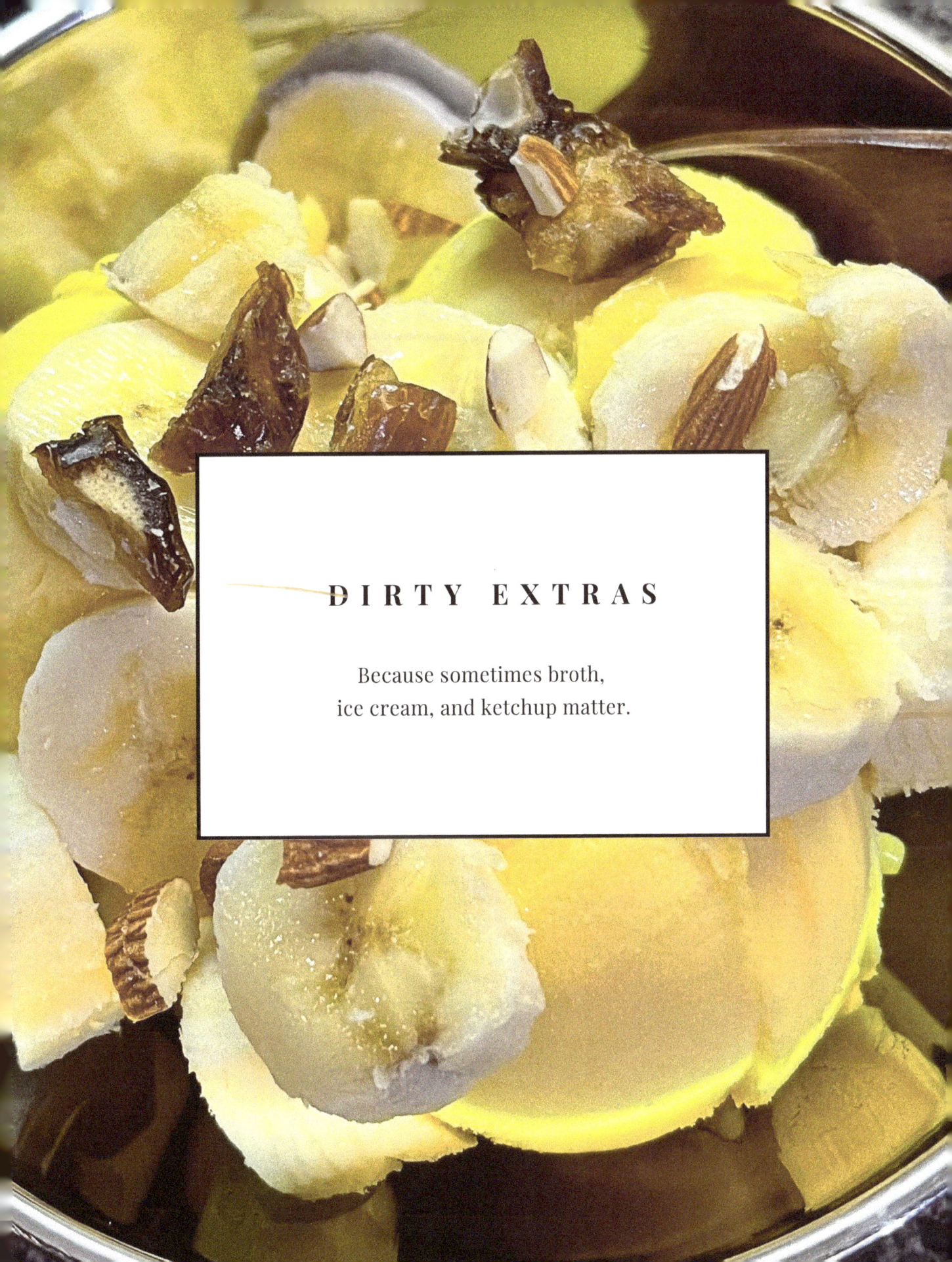

DIRTY EXTRAS

Because sometimes broth,
ice cream, and ketchup matter.

DIRTY EXTRAS

- Easy-Peel Hard-Boiled Eggs
- Homemade Chicken Broth
- Roasted Butternut Squash
- Mashed Potatoes
- Fresh Breakfast Potatoes
- Roasted Sweet Potato Rounds
- Cauliflower Mushroom Risotto
- Coleslaw
- Ketchup
- Cocktail Sauce
- Memphis-style BBQ Sauce
- Chicken & Rib BBQ Sauce
- Yum Yum Fusion Sauce
- Zesty Dill Tartar Sauce
- Sweet Balsamic Salad Dressing
- Homestyle Pan Gravy
- Berry Cobbler
- Dirty Date Brownies
- Banana or Pineapple Ice Cream
- Chocolate Avocado Pudding
- Dubai Luxe Chocolate Bowl

EASY-PEEL HARD-BOILED EGGS
MADE IN THE NINJA FOODI MACHINE OR ON THE STOVETOP

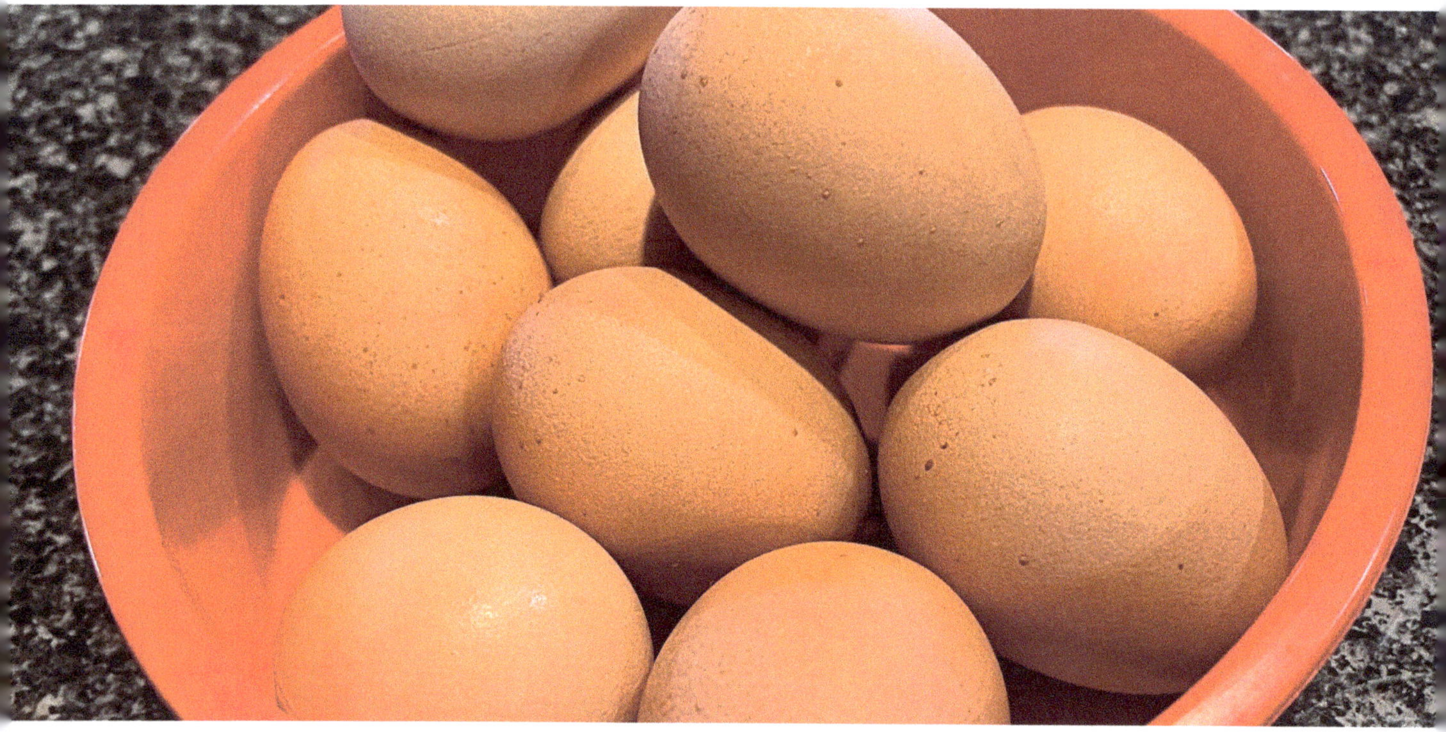

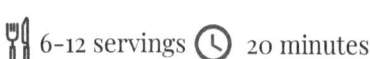

6-12 servings   20 minutes

INGREDIENTS

- 6 to 12 large fresh eggs
- 1 cup water

DIRECTIONS

1. Pour 1 cup of water into the Ninja Foodi inner pot.
2. Place the eggs on a trivet or in a steamer basket inside the pot.
3. Close the lid and set the valve to SEAL.
4. Select the PRESSURE COOK function and set to HIGH for 5 minutes.
5. Once cooking is complete, quick release the pressure.
6. Carefully transfer the eggs to an ice water bath and chill for 5-10 minutes.
7. Gently crack and peel. The shells should come off easily!

Alternative (if you don't have a Ninja Foodi or pressure cooker):
Place the eggs in a saucepan and cover with cold water by about 1 inch. Bring to a boil, then turn off the heat, cover, and let sit for 10-12 minutes. Transfer to an ice water bath for 5-10 minutes before peeling.

> Immediately transfer eggs to an ice water bath for 5 minutes for easy peeling.

HOMEMADE CHICKEN BROTH

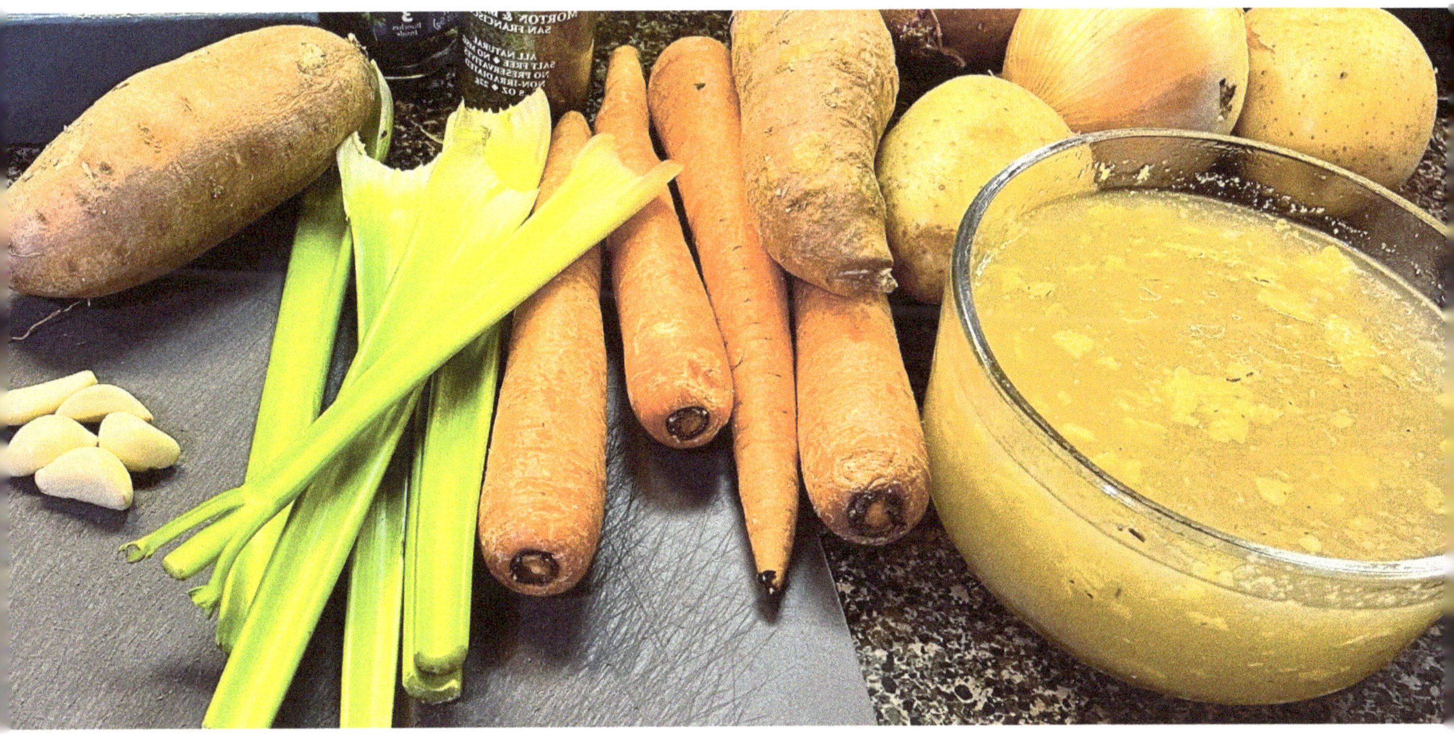

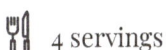 4 servings 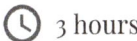 3 hours

INGREDIENTS

- Bones and skin from Oven-Baked Chicken (see Day 3 recipe)
- 8 cups water
- 1 medium onion, quartered
- 2–3 cloves garlic, smashed
- 2 stalks celery, cut into chunks
- 2 carrots, cut into chunks
- 1 bay leaf
- 1 tsp salt (adjust to taste)
- ½ tsp black peppercorns
- Optional: fresh parsley, thyme, or other herbs

DIRECTIONS

1. Place the chicken bones and skin in a large stockpot or Dutch oven.
2. Add the water, onion, garlic, celery, carrots, bay leaf, salt, peppercorns, and any optional herbs.
3. Bring to a boil over medium-high heat, then reduce to a gentle simmer.
4. Simmer uncovered for 2–3 hours, skimming foam as needed and adding water if it reduces too much.
5. Strain the broth through a strainer, discarding solids.
6. Cool and store in the fridge for up to 4 days or freeze for later use.

No vegetables on hand? Just use the bones and skin, and remember a little jiggle when cooled means you pulled out all the good collagen. It's a sign of rich, nourishing broth!

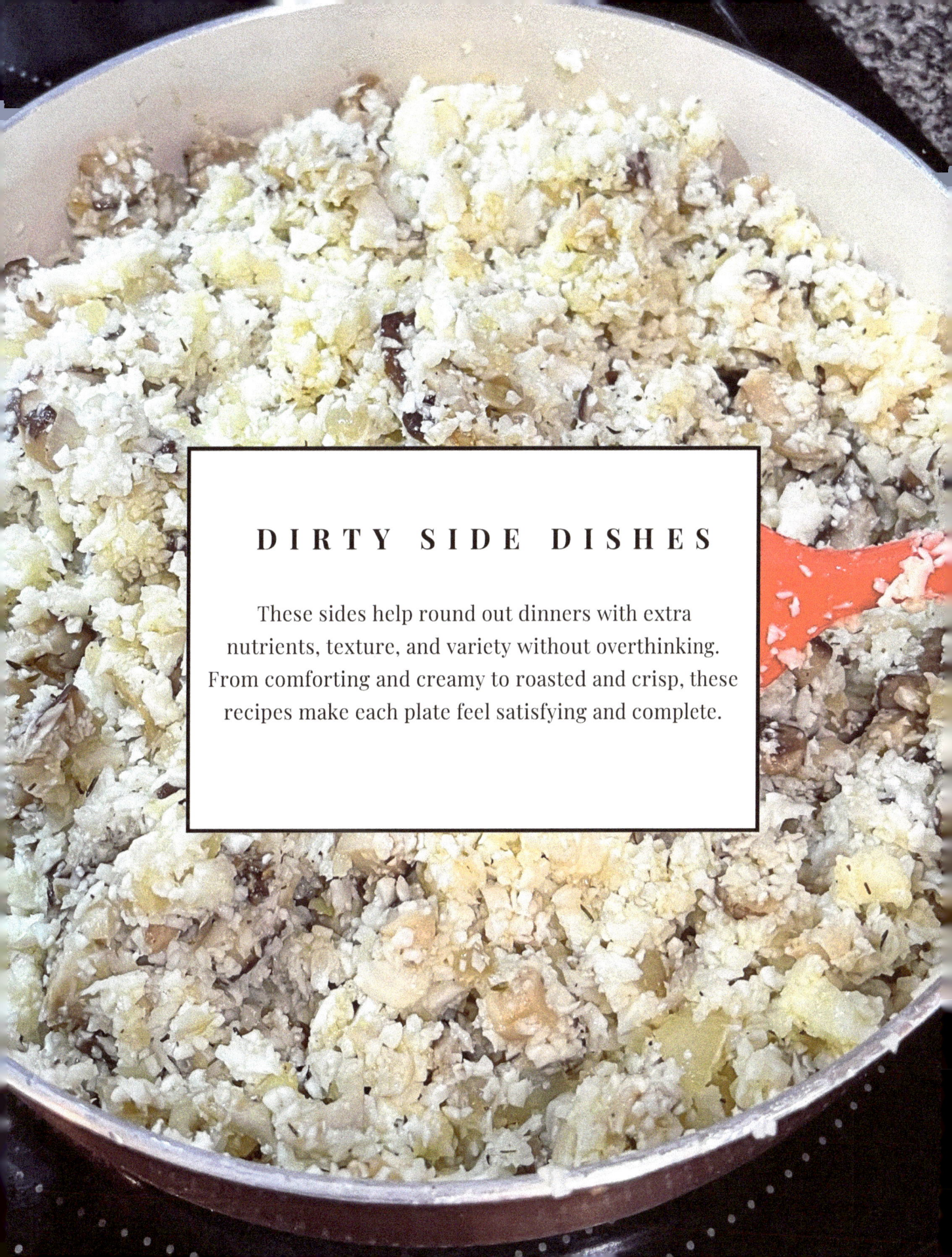

DIRTY SIDE DISHES

These sides help round out dinners with extra nutrients, texture, and variety without overthinking. From comforting and creamy to roasted and crisp, these recipes make each plate feel satisfying and complete.

DIRTY SIDE DISHES

- Roasted Butternut Squash
- Mashed Potatoes
- Fresh Breakfast Potatoes
- Roasted Sweet Potato Rounds
- Cauliflower Mushroom Risotto
- Coleslaw

ROASTED BUTTERNUT SQUASH

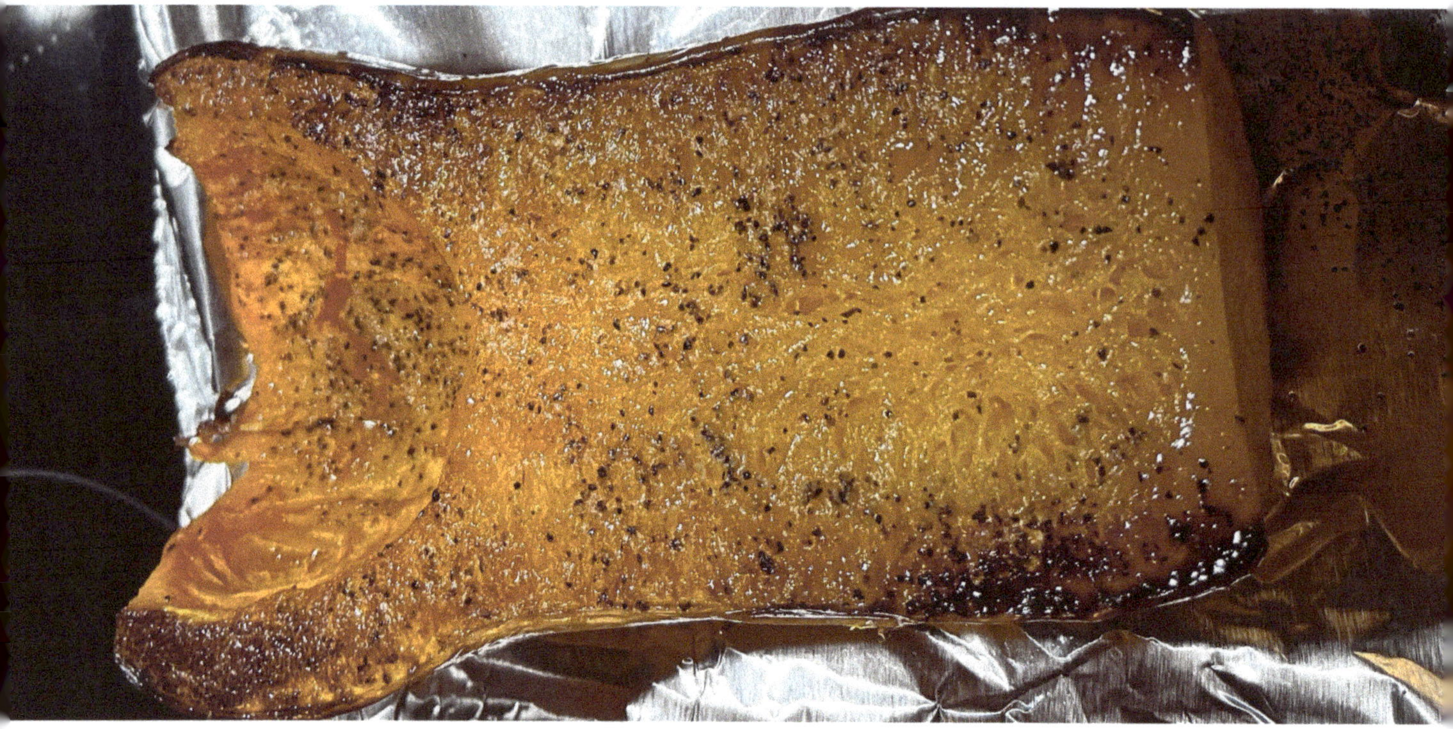

 4 servings 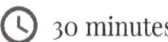 30 minutes

INGREDIENTS

- 1 medium butternut squash
- 1–2 Tbsp avocado or olive oil
- Salt & pepper to taste
- Optional: garlic powder for extra flavor

DIRECTIONS

1. Preheat oven to 400°F.
2. Microwave the whole butternut squash for 2–3 minutes to make it easier to cut. Let it cool slightly.
3. Cut the squash in half lengthwise and scoop out the seeds.
4. Place the halves cut-side down on a parchment-lined baking sheet.
5. Roast for 40–45 minutes until very tender, or roast for 20–25 minutes, scoop out the flesh, cut into cubes, and return to the baking sheet. Roast cubes another 15–20 minutes, stirring once halfway through, until lightly browned.

> The edges of the squash cubes will get golden and caramelized as they roast — those bits are the best part, so don't be afraid of a little browning!

FRESH BREAKFAST POTATOES

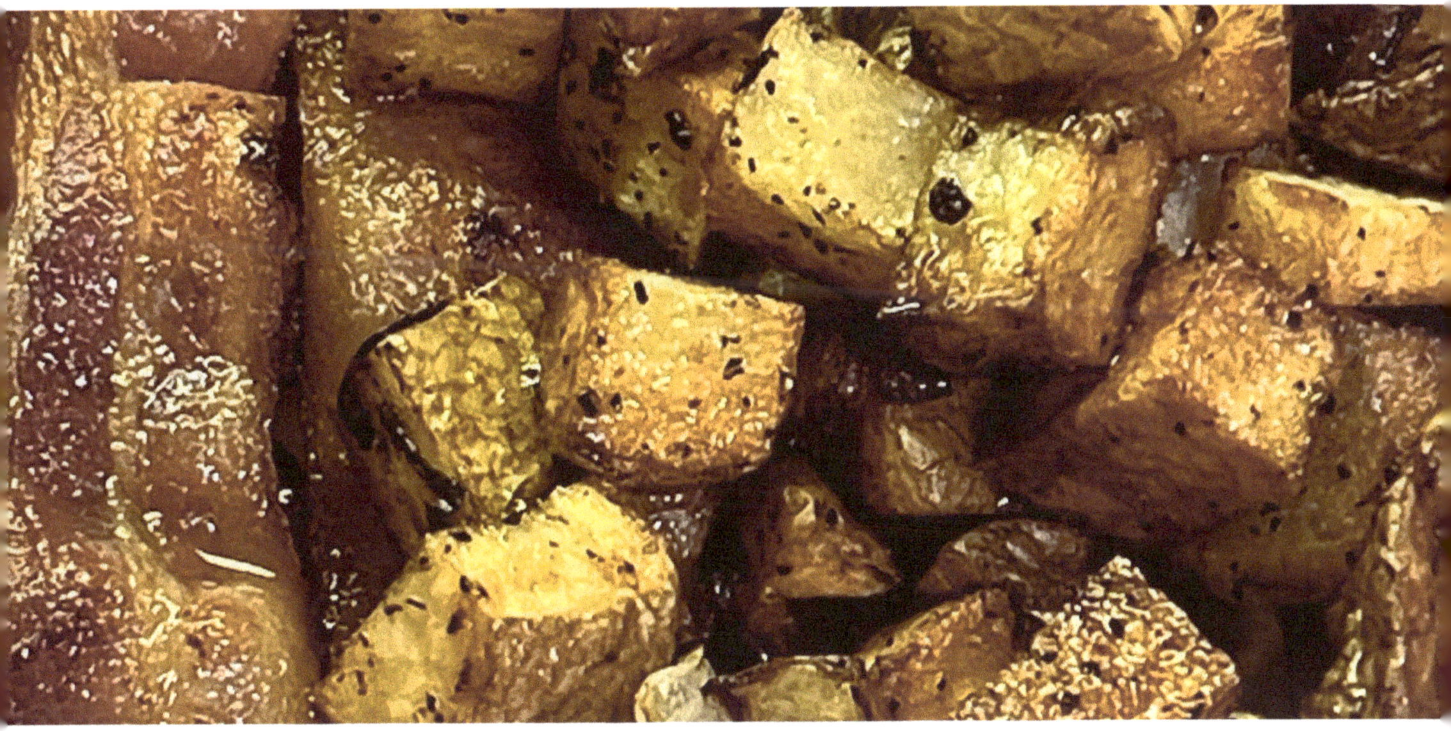

 4 servings  30 minutes

INGREDIENTS

- Avocado or olive oil, for frying
- 2 large russet potatoes, unpeeled and diced
- 1 onion, chopped
- Salt & pepper, to taste

DIRECTIONS

1. Heat a skillet over medium heat and add enough oil to coat the bottom.
2. Add the diced potato and cook, stirring occasionally, until about halfway done and starting to brown.
3. Add the chopped onion and continue cooking, stirring as needed, for about 5 minutes until the potatoes are golden and the onions are browned and softened.
4. Season with salt and pepper to taste.
5. Serve hot.

For extra crispy potatoes, don't stir too often. Let them sit and brown between turns.

ROASTED SWEET POTATO ROUNDS

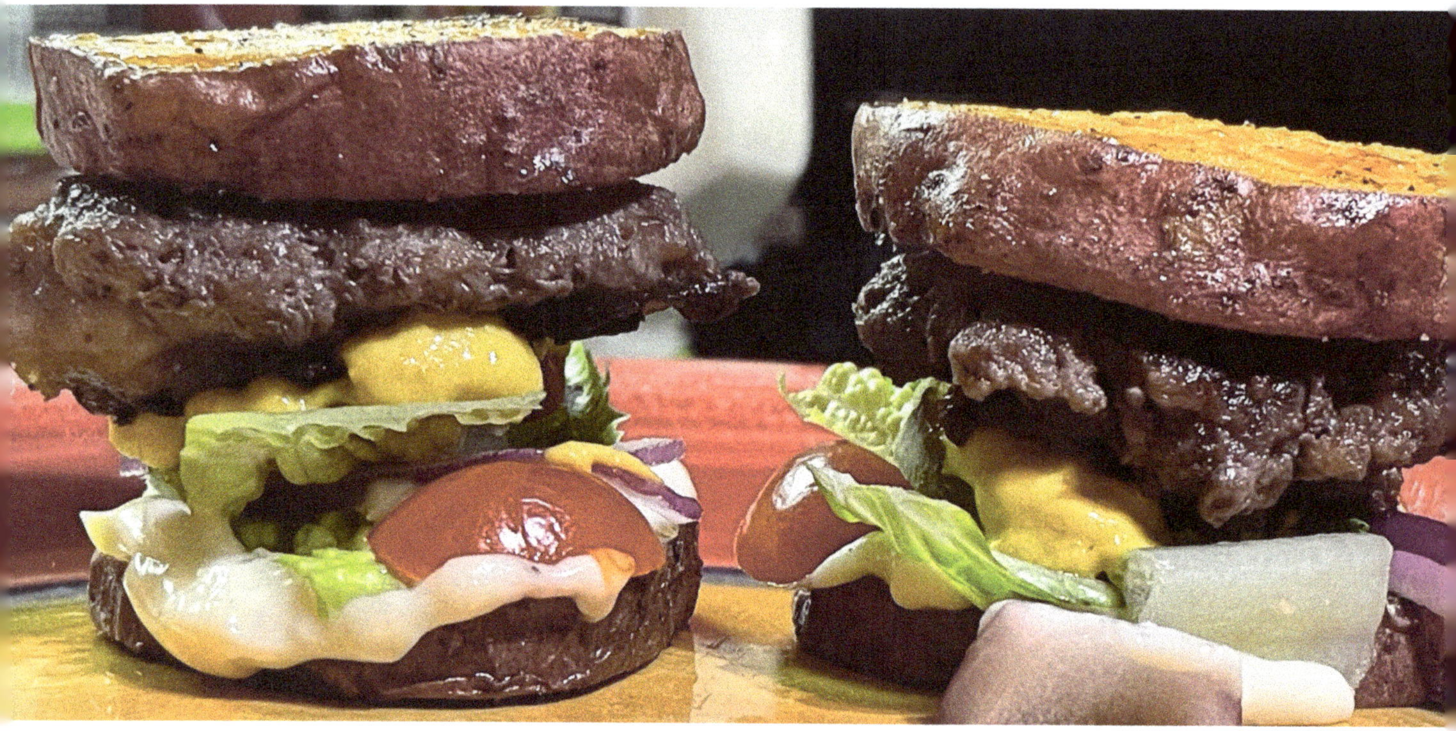

 4 servings 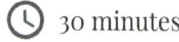 30 minutes

INGREDIENTS

- 2 medium sweet potatoes, scrubbed
- 1-2 Tbsp avocado or olive oil
- Salt & pepper to taste
- Optional: garlic powder or smoked paprika for extra flavor

DIRECTIONS

1. Preheat your oven to 400°F.
2. Slice the sweet potatoes into 1/4 to 1/2 inch thick rounds.
3. Toss the rounds with oil, salt, and any optional seasonings.
4. Arrange in a single layer on a baking sheet.
5. Roast for 25-30 minutes, flipping halfway through, until tender and golden brown on the edges.

Sweet Potato Three Ways
- Eat them sliced just as they are.
- Cube them for easy side dishes.
- Use them as "buns" for burgers: Slice closer to ¼ inch thick so they crisp up more, then roast until the edges are browned and the centers are firm. Let them cool a few minutes before building your burger. They're not as sturdy as bread, but they make a delicious real-food swap that works especially well for sliders or knife-and-fork burgers.

Let the edges get a little browned —
that caramelization brings out the natural sweetness and makes every bite extra good.

MASHED POTATOES

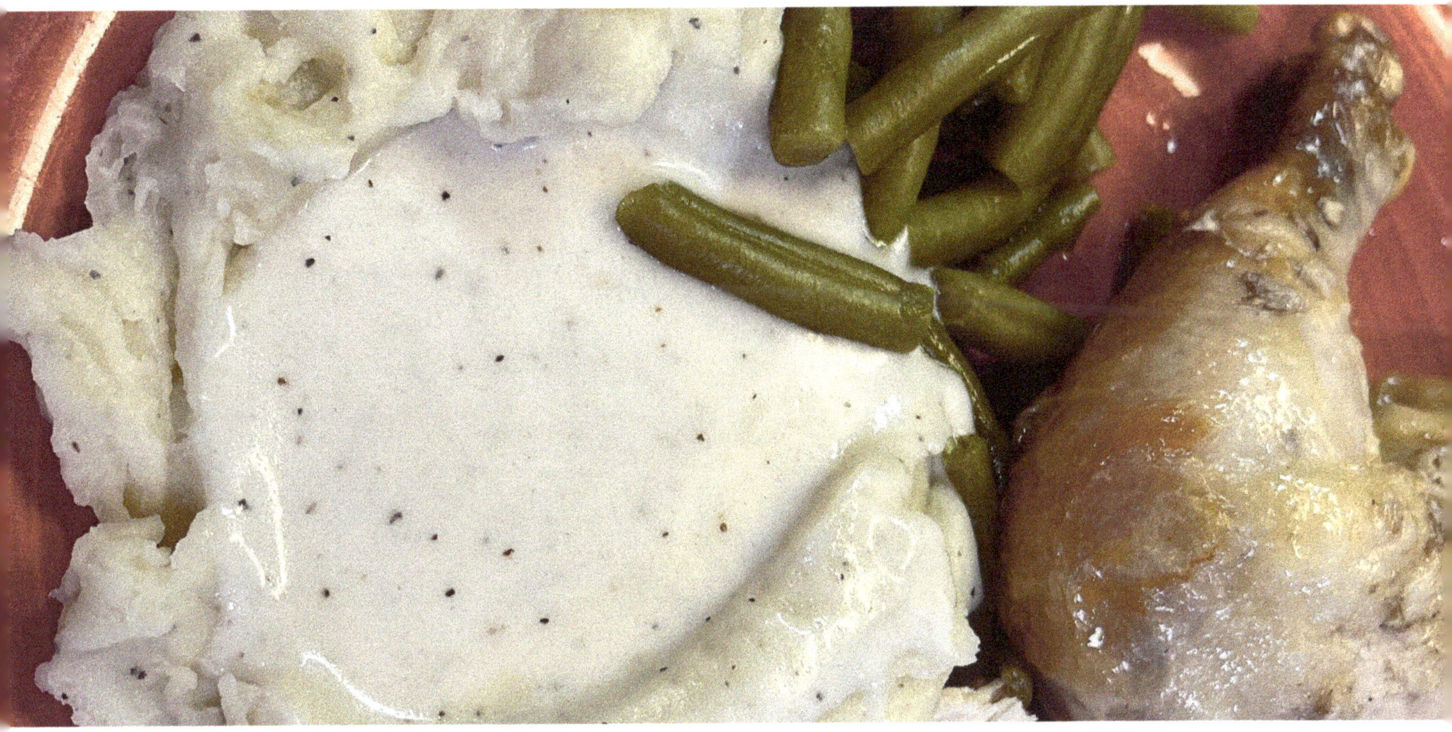

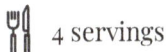 4 servings 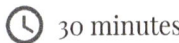 30 minutes

INGREDIENTS

- 2 lbs (about 4 medium) russet or Yukon Gold potatoes, peeled or unpeeled (your choice), cut into chunks
- 2–3 Tbsp ghee (or more to taste)
- ¼ to ½ cup coconut milk (add more as needed for desired creaminess)
- Salt & pepper to taste
- Optional: garlic powder or chopped fresh herbs (like parsley)

DIRECTIONS

1. Place potato chunks in a large pot and cover with cold water. Add a generous pinch of salt.
2. Bring to a boil over medium-high heat, then reduce heat and simmer until potatoes are fork-tender, about 15–20 minutes.
3. Drain the potatoes well and return them to the pot.
4. Add ghee and a splash of coconut milk. Mash until smooth, adding more coconut milk as needed to reach your preferred texture. If leaving skins on, mash to your preferred consistency.
5. Taste and season with salt, pepper and any optional add-ins like garlic powder.
6. Serve hot, topped with extra ghee or fresh herbs if desired.

These potatoes are easy to make your own. Keep them rustic with the skins on, or mash them smooth and creamy. Either way, don't skip tasting as you go so the seasoning is just right!

CAULIFLOWER MUSHROOM RISOTTO

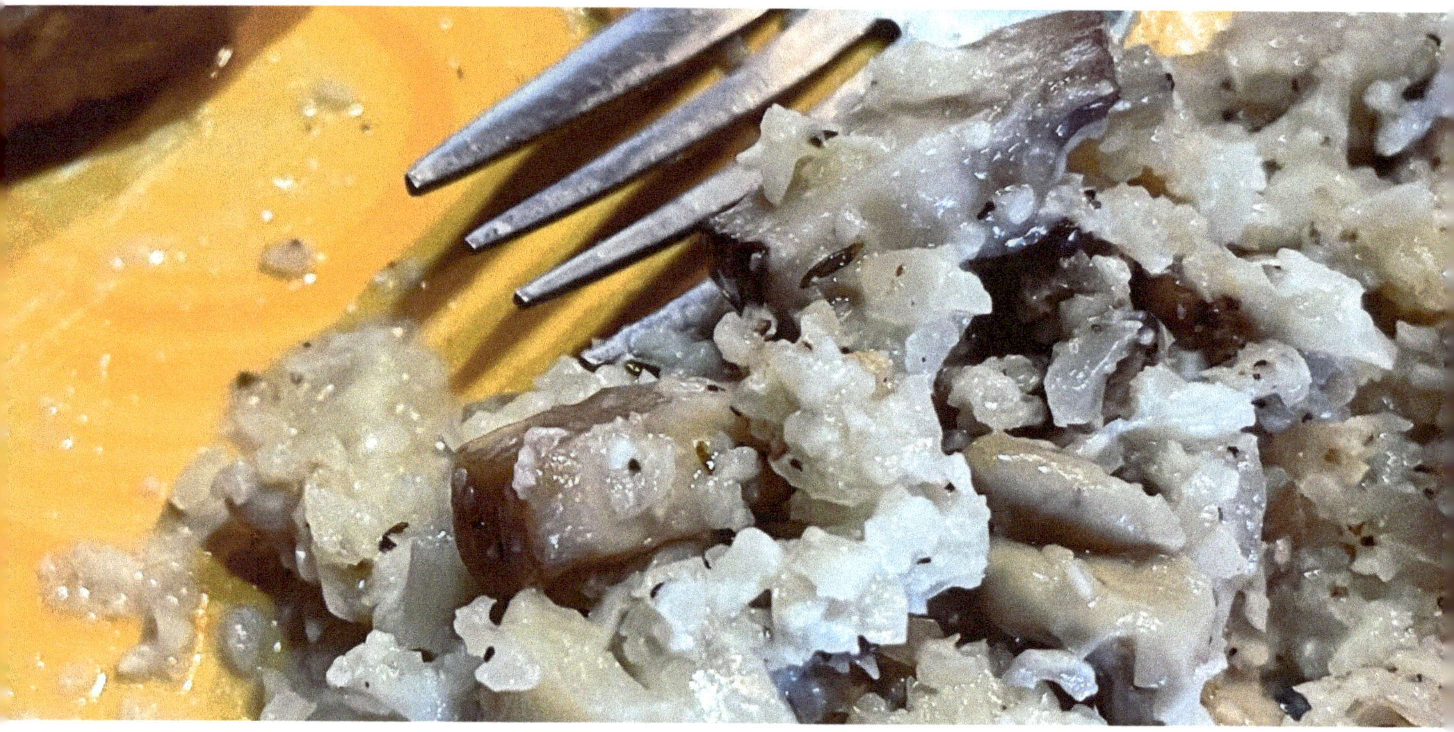

 4 servings 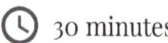 30 minutes

INGREDIENTS

- 1 Tbsp avocado or olive oil
- 8 oz mushrooms, sliced
- 3 cups riced cauliflower
- 2 cloves garlic, minced
- ½ cup chicken or vegetable broth
- ¼ cup coconut milk
- 1 Tbsp coconut aminos (optional, for extra savory flavor)
- Salt & pepper, to taste
- Optional: fresh parsley for garnish

DIRECTIONS

1. Heat the oil in a skillet over medium heat.
2. Add the sliced mushrooms and cook until browned and tender, about 5–7 minutes.
3. Stir in the garlic and cook for 30 seconds until fragrant.
4. Add the riced cauliflower and stir to combine.
5. Pour in the broth and coconut aminos (if using). Stir well.
6. Cook, stirring occasionally, for 6–8 minutes or until the cauliflower is tender and most of the liquid has absorbed.
7. Stir in the coconut milk and let it warm through, coating the cauliflower mixture.
8. Season with salt and pepper to taste.
9. Garnish with fresh parsley, if desired, and serve warm.

Want deeper flavor? Use a mix of mushrooms (like cremini and shiitake) or add a sprinkle of nutritional yeast for a cheesy vibe without the cheese.

COLESLAW

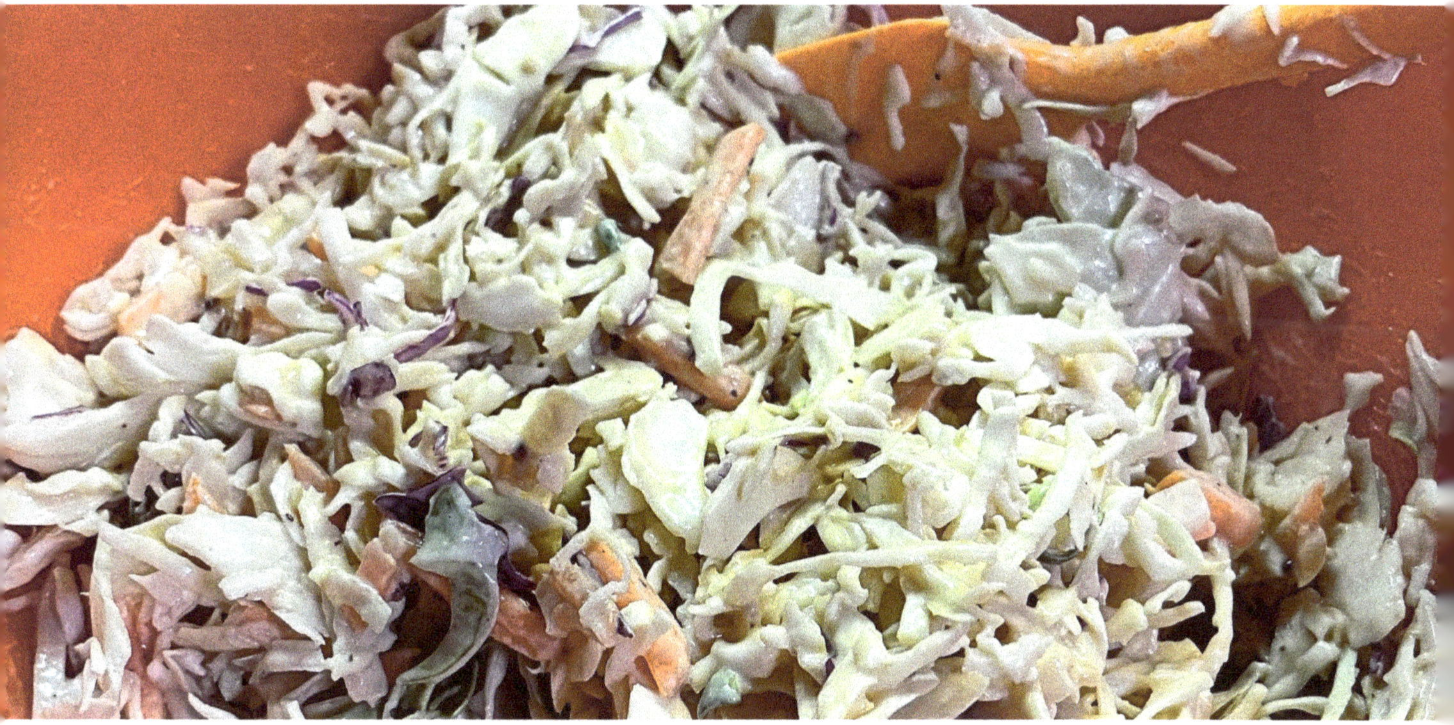

 4 servings 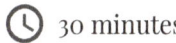 30 minutes

INGREDIENTS

- 1 cup avocado oil mayonnaise
- 2 Tbsp apple cider vinegar
- 1 Tbsp lemon juice
- 1 Tbsp coconut aminos, or more to taste
- 2 Tbsp Dijon mustard
- 1–3 Tbsp date syrup, as desired
- Salt & pepper to taste
- 4–6 cups shredded cabbage and carrots
- ¼ cup finely diced onion
- Optional: pinch of celery seed

DIRECTIONS

1. Whisk together mayo, apple cider vinegar, lemon juice, coconut aminos, Dijon, salt, pepper, and date syrup in a small bowl.
2. Toss shredded cabbage, carrots, and diced onion with dressing until well coated.
3. Sprinkle celery seed on top if using.
4. Chill for at least 30 minutes before serving for best flavor.

Make it ahead—it gets even better after a few hours in the fridge. Serve it with ribs, wings, or anything that needs a little crisp and cool on the side.

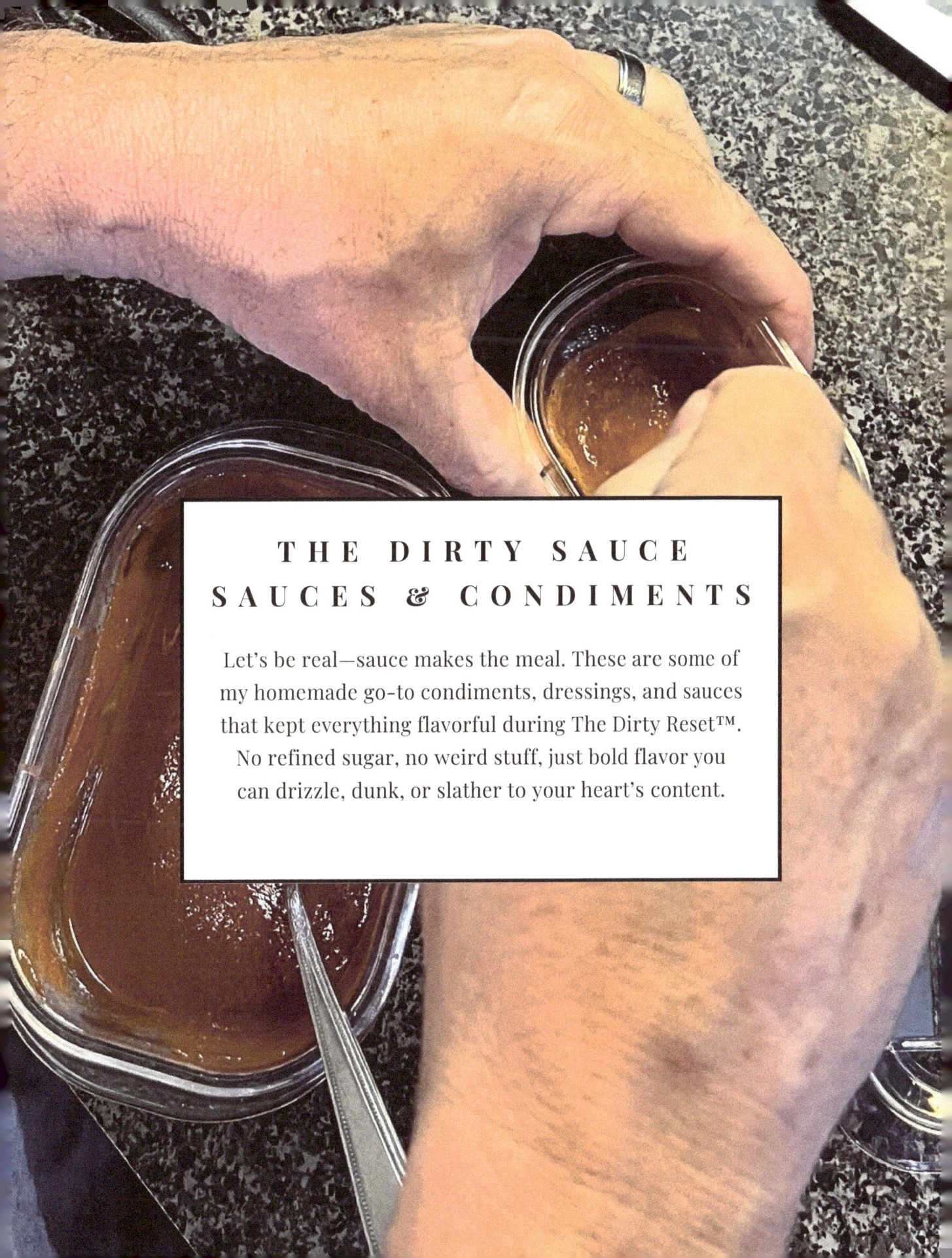

THE DIRTY SAUCE
SAUCES & CONDIMENTS

Let's be real—sauce makes the meal. These are some of my homemade go-to condiments, dressings, and sauces that kept everything flavorful during The Dirty Reset™. No refined sugar, no weird stuff, just bold flavor you can drizzle, dunk, or slather to your heart's content.

THE DIRTY SAUCE
SAUCES & CONDIMENTS

- Ketchup
- Cocktail Sauce
- Memphis-style BBQ Sauce
- Chicken & Rib BBQ Sauce
- Yum Yum Fusion Sauce
- Zesty Dill Tartar Sauce
- Sweet Balsamic Salad Dressing
- Homestyle Pan Gravy

KETCHUP

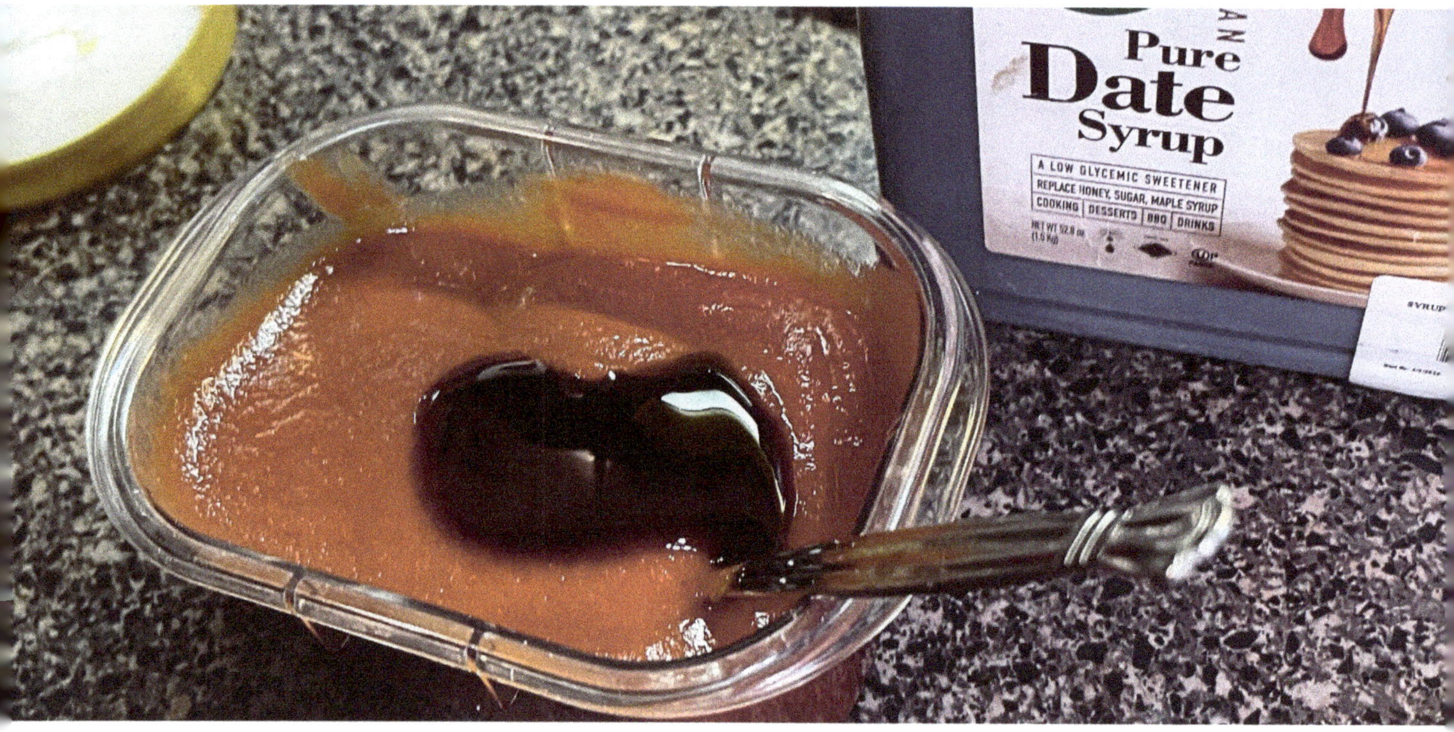

12 servings   5 minutes

INGREDIENTS

- 1 can (6 oz) tomato paste
- 2 Tbsp apple cider vinegar
- 1 Tbsp lemon juice
- 1 Tbsp date syrup, or to taste
- ½ tsp garlic powder
- ½ tsp onion powder
- ½ tsp salt
- ¼ tsp smoked paprika (optional)
- ¼–½ cup water (adjust to desired consistency)

DIRECTIONS

1. In a medium bowl, whisk together tomato paste, apple cider vinegar, lemon juice, and date syrup.
2. Add garlic powder, onion powder, salt, and smoked paprika if using.
3. Slowly whisk in water a little at a time until you reach your desired ketchup consistency.
4. Taste and adjust seasoning or sweetness as needed.
5. Store in an airtight container in the fridge for up to one week.

Adjust the sweetness and tang by adding more date syrup or vinegar to suit your taste.

COCKTAIL SAUCE

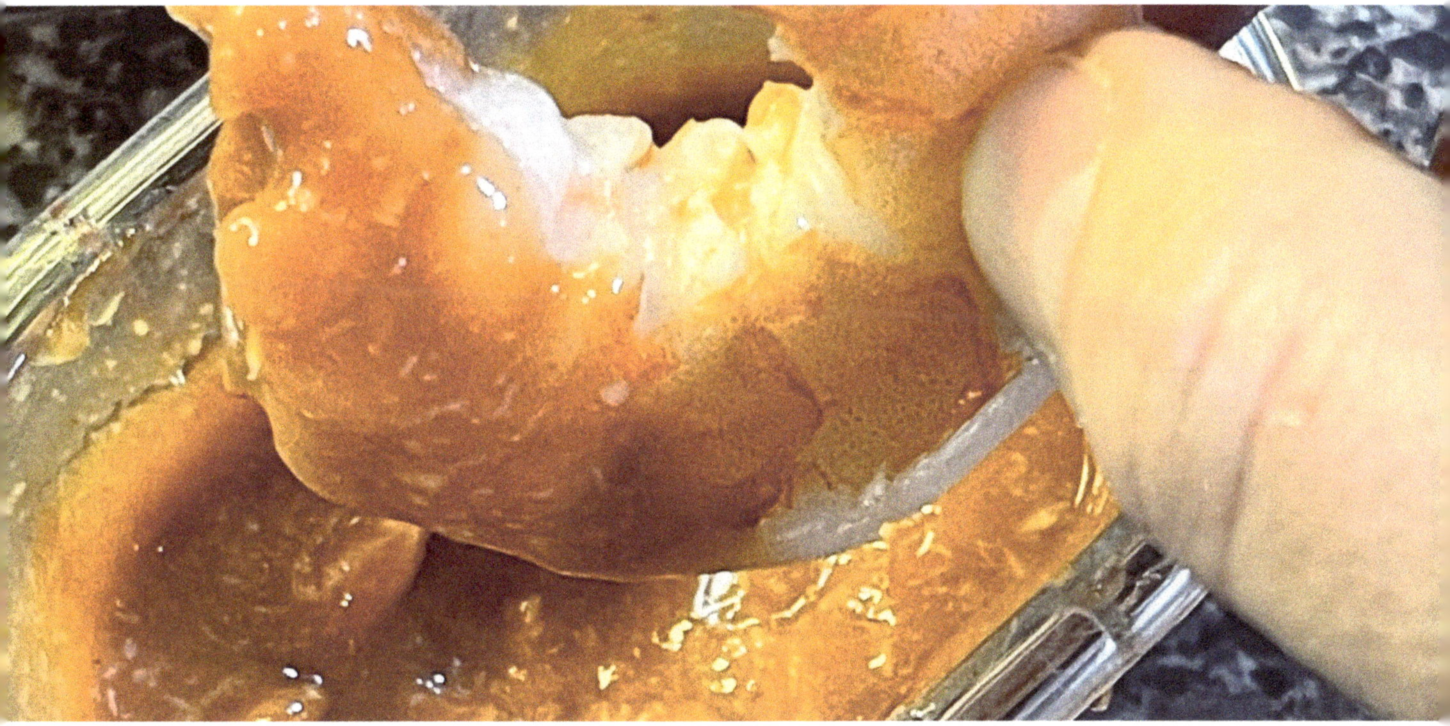

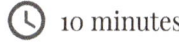 8 servings 10 minutes

INGREDIENTS

- 1 cup Homemade Ketchup (see The Dirty Reset™ recipe)
- 2–2½ Tbsp prepared horseradish

DIRECTIONS

1. In a bowl, combine the ketchup and horseradish.
2. Stir well until fully mixed.
3. Chill for at least 15 minutes before serving.

This Dirty Reset™ cocktail sauce is quick, simple, and packed with flavor. With only two ingredients, it's the perfect dip for seafood.

MEMPHIS-STYLE BBQ SAUCE

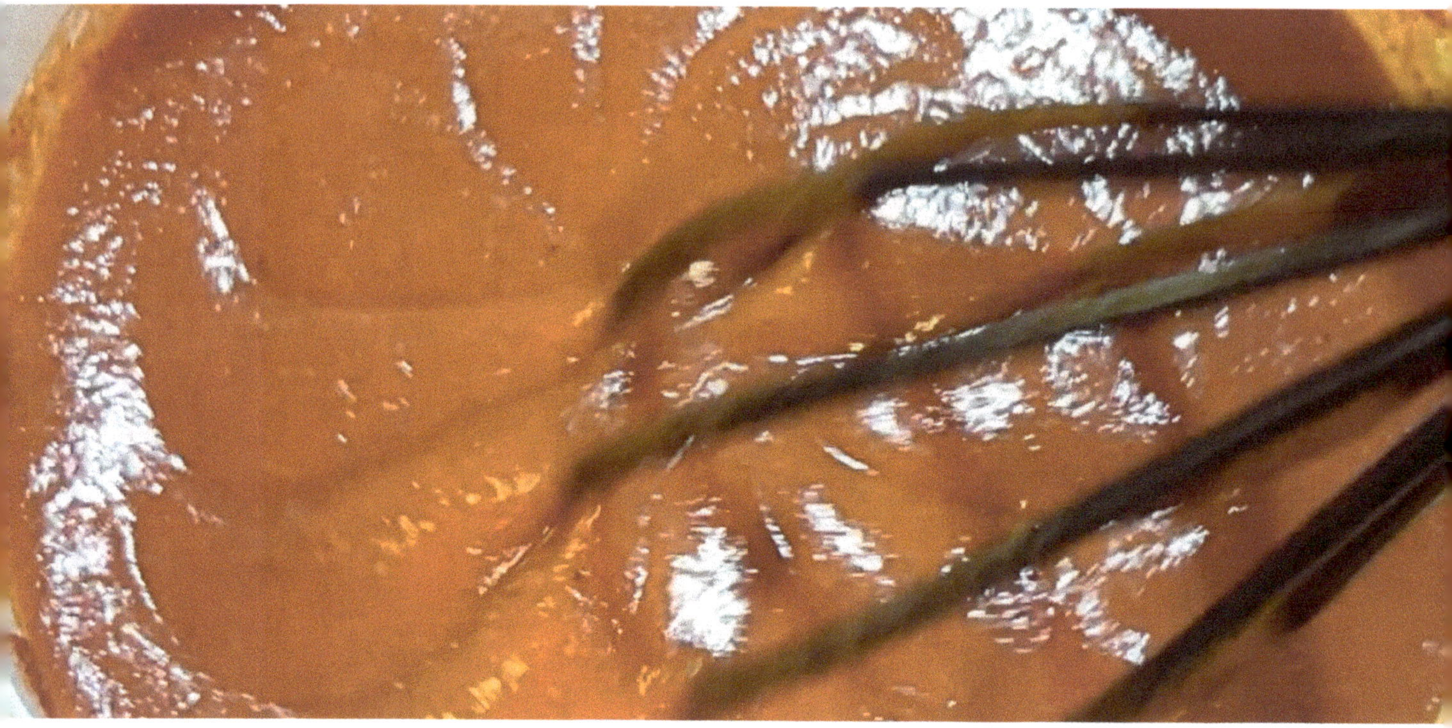

 8 servings 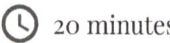 20 minutes

INGREDIENTS

- 1 can (8 oz) tomato sauce
- ¼ cup apple cider vinegar
- 2 Tbsp date syrup, or to taste
- 1 Tbsp Dijon mustard
- 1 tsp garlic powder
- 1 tsp onion powder
- ½ tsp smoked paprika
- ½ tsp salt
- ½ tsp pepper
- Optional: pinch of cayenne for heat

DIRECTIONS

1. Combine all ingredients in a saucepan over medium heat.
2. Stir well and bring to a simmer.
3. Lower heat and let it cook for 15–20 minutes, stirring occasionally, until thickened.
4. Taste and adjust seasoning as needed. Cool before storing in an airtight container in the fridge.

> Use this version when you want a tangier, sharper, more spice-forward sauce. It strikes a balance of tangy, sweet, and spicy. Taste as you go and adjust with extra date syrup or vinegar as needed.

CHICKEN & RIB BBQ SAUCE

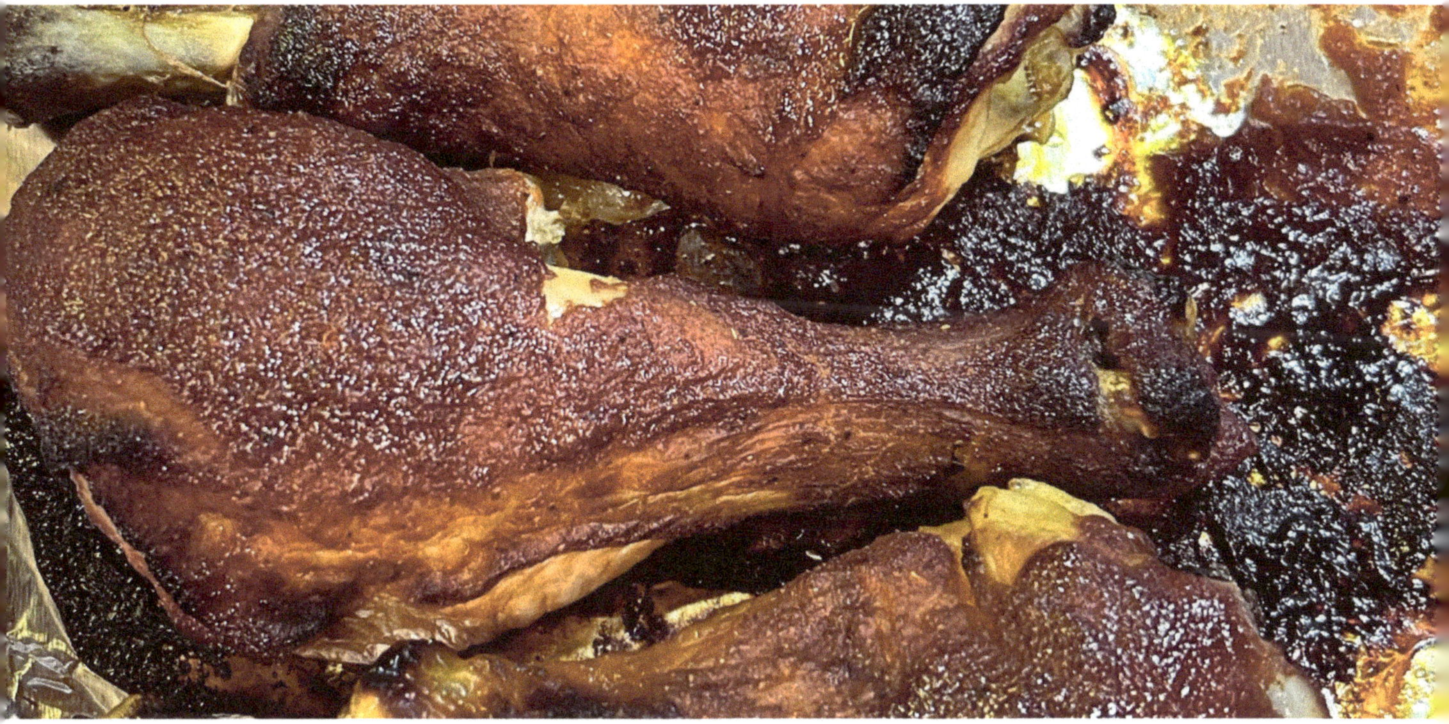

 4 servings 20 minutes

INGREDIENTS

- 1 can (8 oz) tomato sauce
- 2 Tbsp date syrup
- 2 Tbsp apple cider vinegar
- 1 Tbsp coconut aminos
- 1 Tbsp Dijon mustard
- 1 tsp smoked paprika
- ½ tsp garlic powder
- ½ tsp onion powder
- ¼ tsp ground cumin
- ¼ tsp pepper
- ¼ tsp salt
- Optional: pinch cayenne for heat or ½ tsp chipotle powder for smoky spice

DIRECTIONS

1. Add all ingredients to a small saucepan.
2. Stir well and bring to a simmer over medium heat.
3. Reduce heat to low and let simmer 15–20 minutes, stirring occasionally, until thickened.
4. Taste and adjust sweetness or spice to your liking.
5. Let cool slightly, then use as a brush-on sauce for grilled or oven-baked chicken or ribs. You can also use it as a marinade!

> Use this version for a milder, smokier sauce that's a little sweeter and more savory. Brush it on during the last few minutes of grilling, or serve on the side for dipping.

YUM YUM FUSION SAUCE

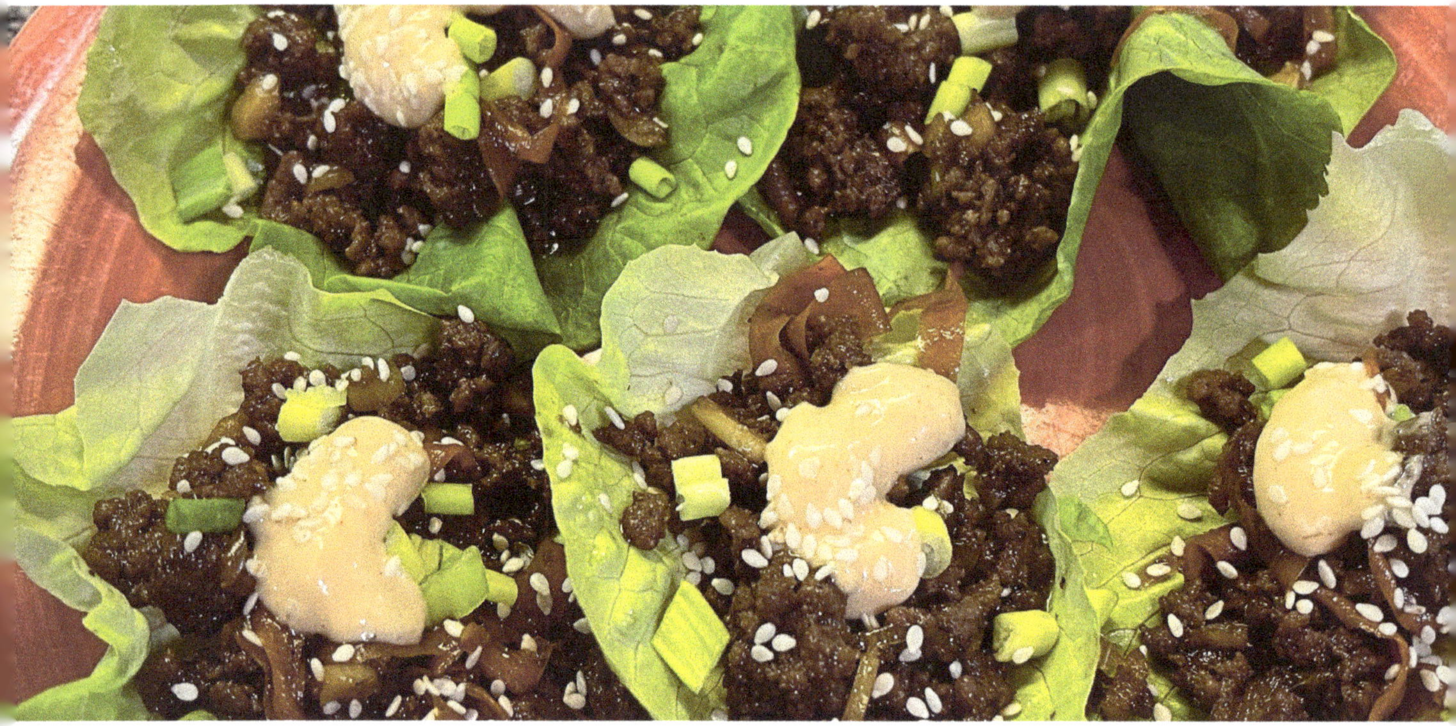

 4 servings 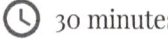 30 minutes

INGREDIENTS

- ¼ cup coconut cream
- 1 Tbsp tomato paste (or The Dirty Reset™ Ketchup)
- 1 Tbsp coconut aminos
- 1 tsp apple cider vinegar
- ½ tsp garlic powder
- ½ tsp onion powder
- 1 tsp smoked paprika
- 1 tsp date syrup
- ¼ tsp Dijon mustard
- ¼ tsp toasted sesame oil
- Optional: splash of water to thin

DIRECTIONS

1. Whisk all ingredients together in a bowl until smooth and creamy.
2. Add a splash of water if you prefer a thinner sauce for drizzling.
3. Taste and adjust vinegar, sweetness, or sesame oil as needed.
4. Chill for 15–30 minutes before serving to let the flavors blend.

This sauce has a rich, slightly nutty flavor, almost like peanut sauce, but it contains no peanuts. It's a great alternative for anyone avoiding them.

ZESTY DILL TARTAR SAUCE

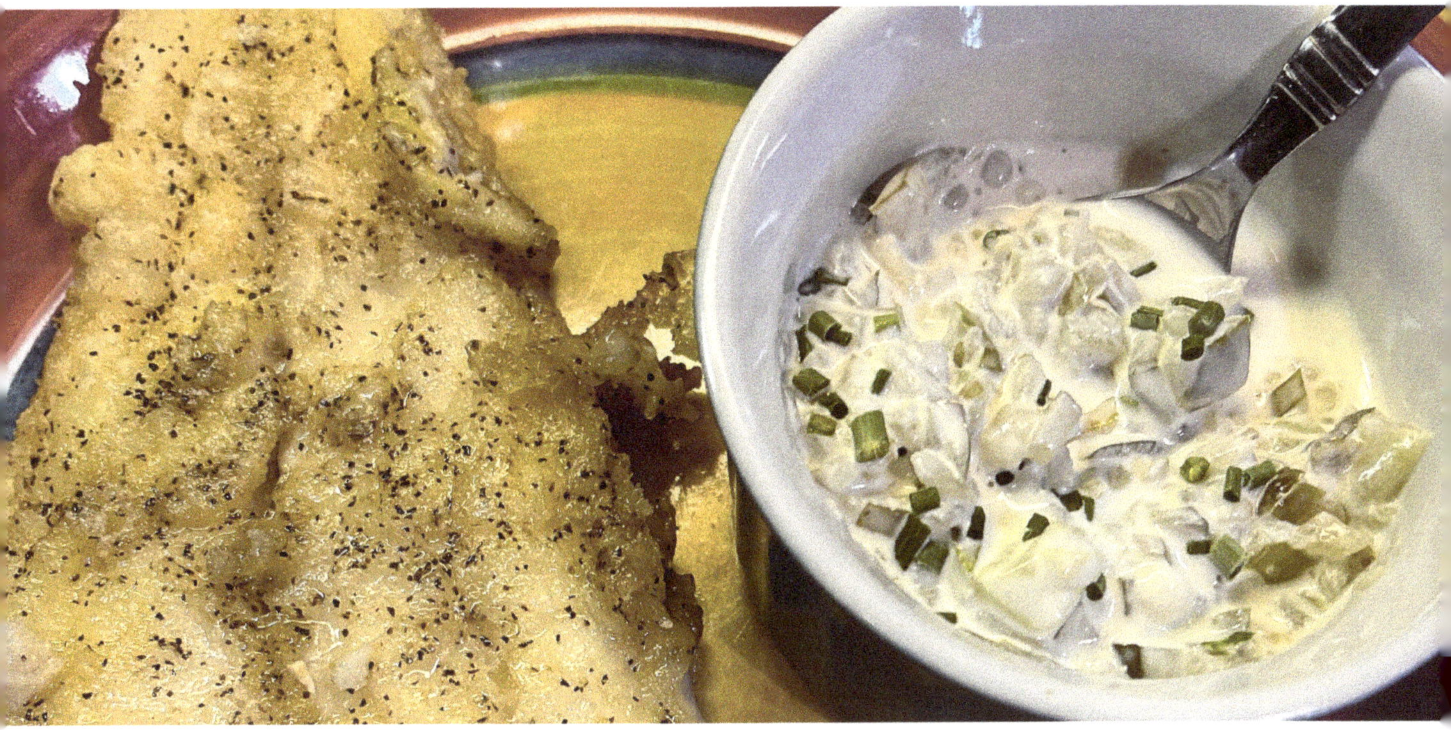

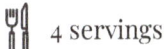 4 servings 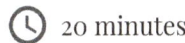 20 minutes

INGREDIENTS

- ½ cup avocado oil mayonnaise
- 1 Tbsp pickle juice or lemon juice (to taste)
- ¼ cup minced dill pickles or no-sugar-added dill relish

DIRECTIONS

1. In a small bowl, combine the avocado mayo with pickle juice or lemon juice.
2. Stir in the minced dill pickles or relish.
3. Mix until well combined and creamy.
4. Taste and adjust acidity or saltiness as needed.
5. Chill for 10–15 minutes before serving for best flavor.

> For extra flavor, stir in a pinch of garlic powder, fresh dill, or a splash of coconut aminos. Let the sauce chill for at least 10 minutes before serving to help the flavors blend.

SWEET BALSAMIC SALAD DRESSING

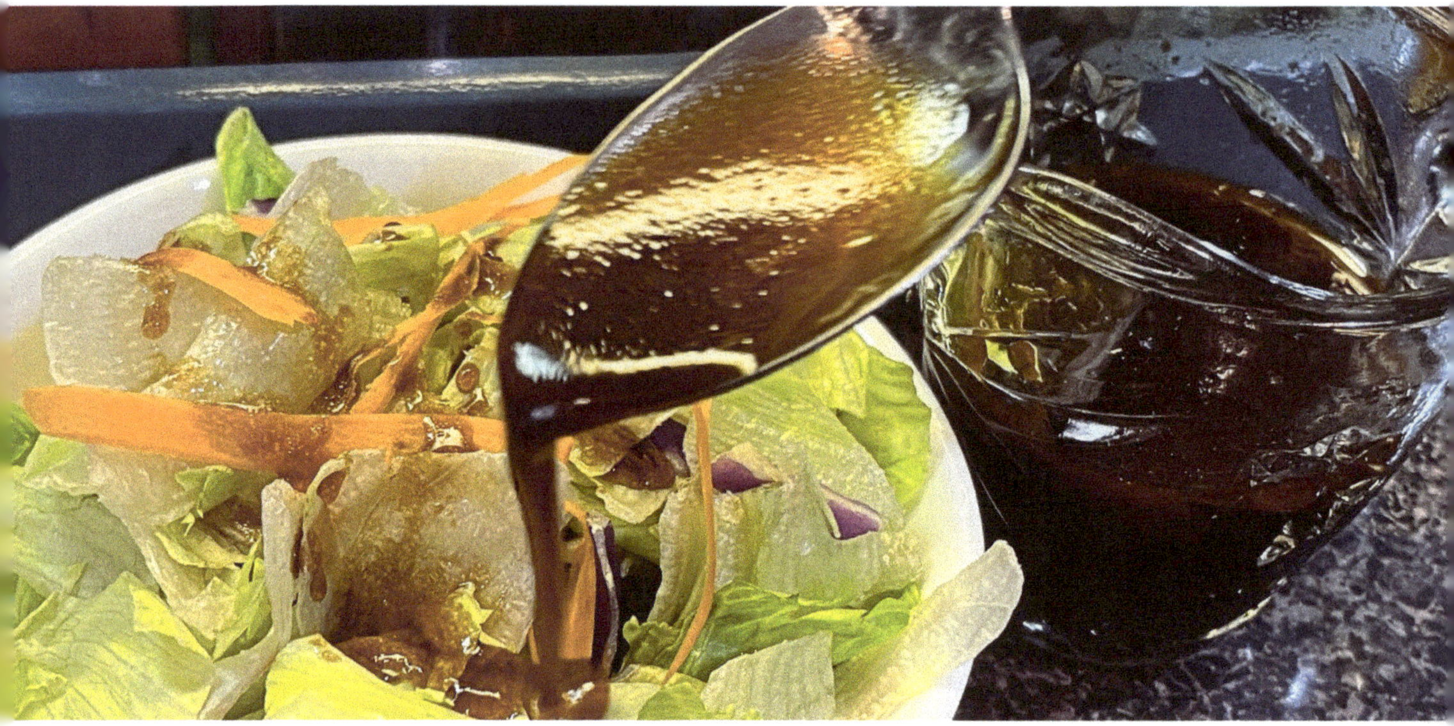

 4 servings 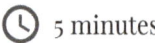 5 minutes

INGREDIENTS

- ¼ cup olive oil
- 2 Tbsp balsamic vinegar
- Date syrup, to taste (start with 1 tsp and adjust as needed)

DIRECTIONS

1. In a small bowl or jar, combine the olive oil and balsamic vinegar.
2. Add date syrup a little at a time, tasting as you go, until it reaches your desired level of sweetness.
3. Whisk or shake vigorously until well combined.

Shake or whisk well before serving. Taste and adjust sweetness or tang as needed. This dressing also works well as a marinade for chicken or vegetables.

HOMESTYLE PAN GRAVY

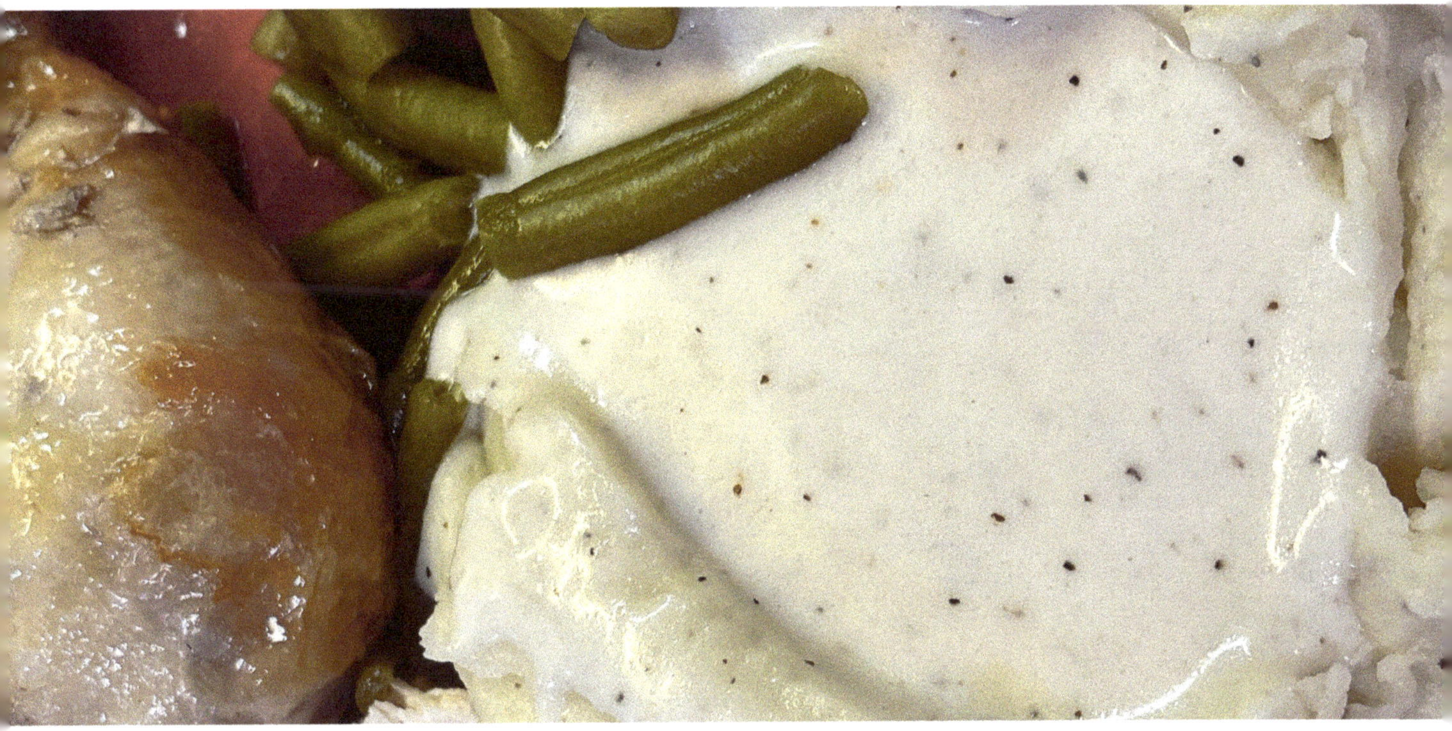

 4 servings   15 minutes

INGREDIENTS

- ¼ cup pan drippings from Oven-Baked Chicken (see Day 3 for recipe), strained if necessary (or supplement with chicken broth if needed)
- 2 cups full-fat coconut milk
- 1 Tbsp tapioca flour
- ¼ cup cold water (for slurry)
- Salt & pepper to taste

DIRECTIONS

1. In a medium saucepan over medium heat, warm the chicken pan drippings. If you don't have enough drippings, add a splash of chicken broth (see Dirty Extras section for recipe).
2. Pour in the coconut milk and whisk until fully combined with the drippings.
3. Stir in salt and pepper to taste. Keep seasoning light at first. You can adjust later.
4. In a small bowl, mix tapioca flour with cold water to make a smooth slurry. Slowly whisk this slurry into the hot coconut mixture.
5. Reduce heat to low and stir continuously for 5–10 minutes, until the gravy thickens to your desired consistency.
6. Adjust seasoning before serving over mashed potatoes, chicken, or vegetables.

For thicker gravy: Simmer the full 10 minutes, whisking often.
For a looser gravy: Stop once it coats the back of a spoon.

> Rich, savory, and perfectly smooth, this gravy is a simple way to turn any roast chicken dinner into pure comfort. Thickened just enough to coat each bite, it's a quick classic you'll want on repeat.

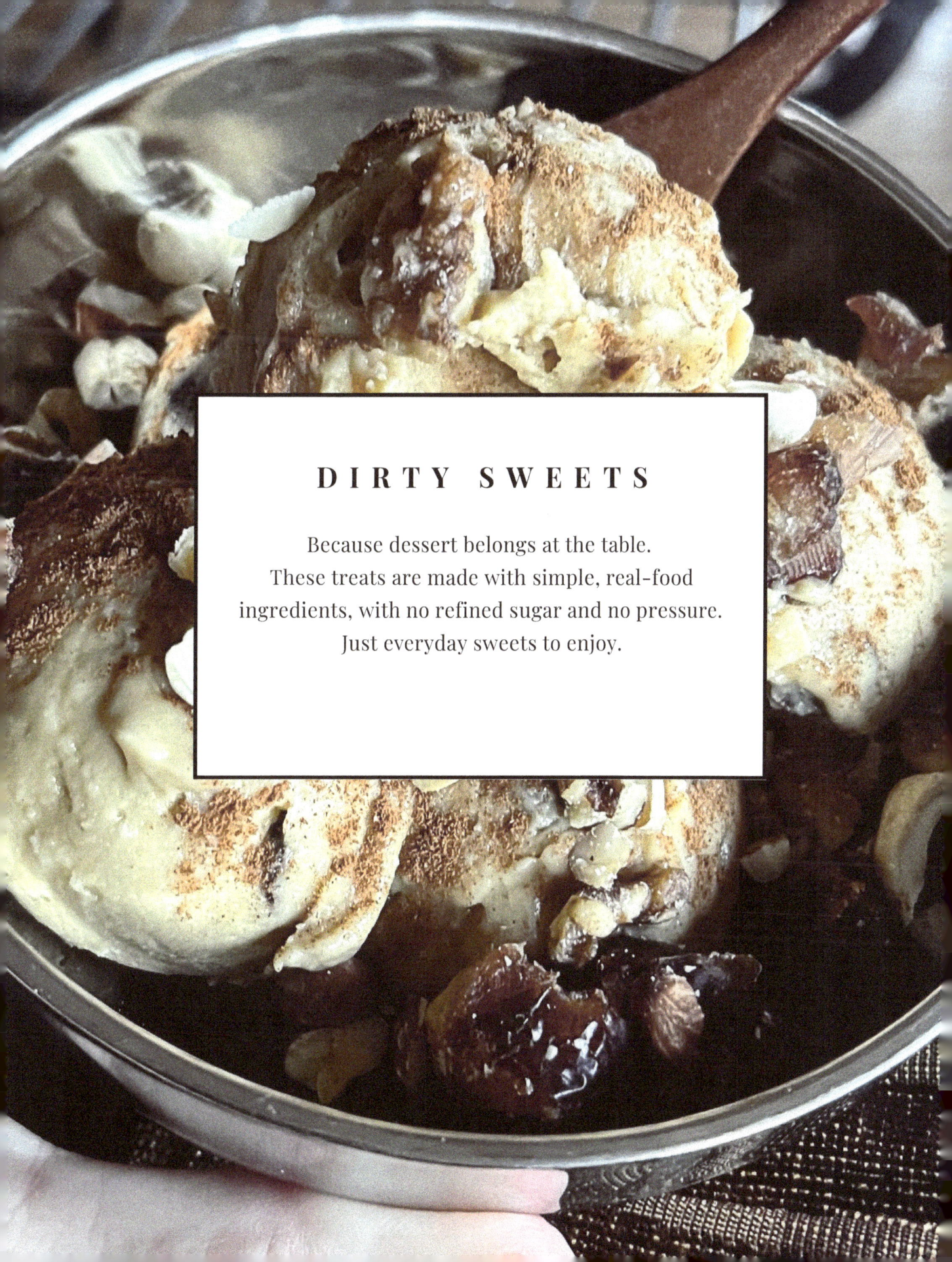

DIRTY SWEETS

Because dessert belongs at the table.
These treats are made with simple, real-food ingredients, with no refined sugar and no pressure.
Just everyday sweets to enjoy.

DIRTY SWEETS

- Berry Cobbler
- Dirty Date Brownies
- Banana or Pineapple Ice Cream
- Chocolate Avocado Pudding
- Dubai Luxe Chocolate Bowl

BERRY COBBLER

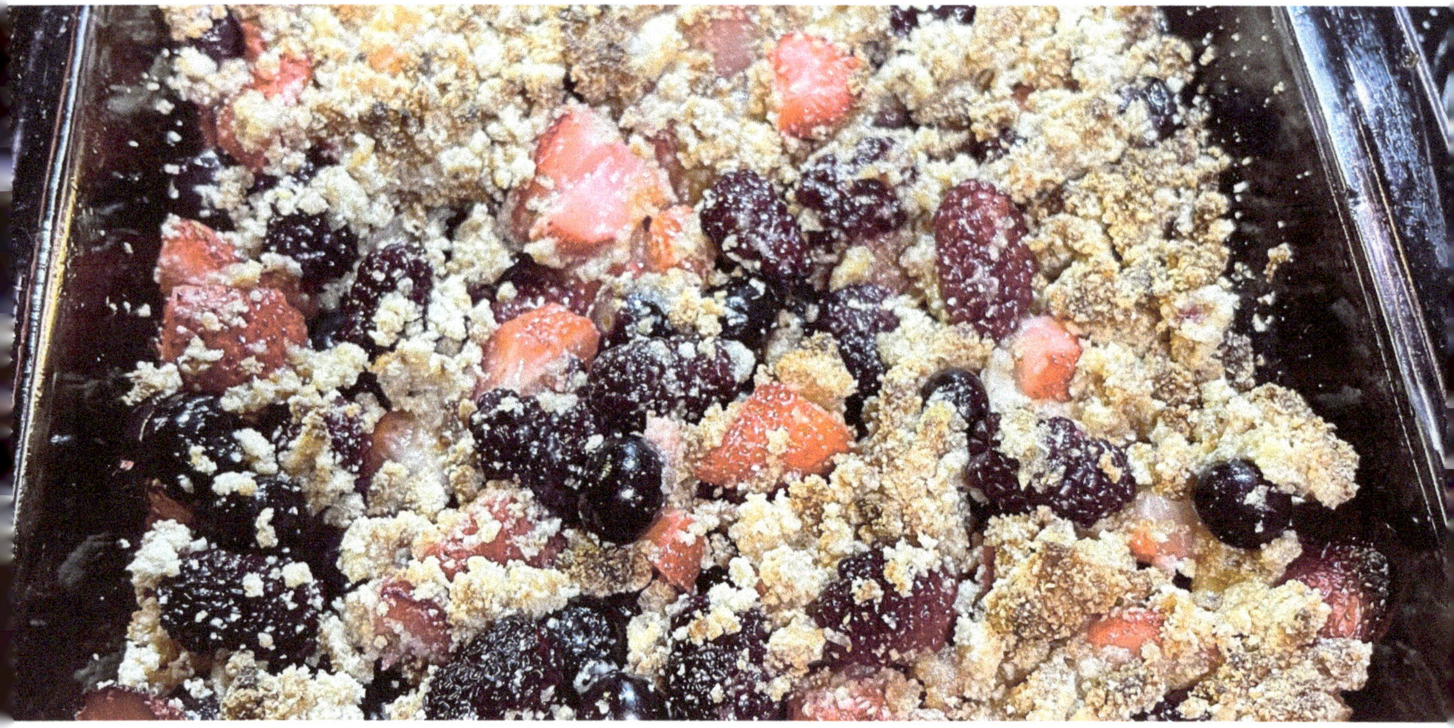

 6 servings 30 minutes

INGREDIENTS

Berry Filling
- 4 cups mixed berries, fresh or frozen
- 2 Tbsp date syrup, or more to taste
- 1 tsp lemon juice
- 1 Tbsp tapioca flour (for thickening)

Almond Flour Topping
- 1 cup almond flour
- 2 Tbsp coconut oil or ghee, melted
- 1 Tbsp date syrup
- ½ tsp cinnamon
- Pinch of salt

DIRECTIONS

1. Preheat oven to 350°F.
2. In a mixing bowl, toss the berries with date syrup, lemon juice, and tapioca flour.
3. Spread the mixture evenly in a small baking dish, about 8×8 or similar.
4. In a separate bowl, mix almond flour, melted coconut oil or ghee, date syrup, cinnamon, and salt until a crumbly dough forms.
5. Sprinkle the topping evenly over the berry mixture.
6. Bake for 25-30 minutes, or until the topping is golden and the berries are bubbling.
7. Let cool slightly before serving.

Let the cobbler cool for at least 10 minutes before serving so the filling can thicken. Serve warm on its own or with coconut cream for an extra treat.

DIRTY DATE BROWNIES

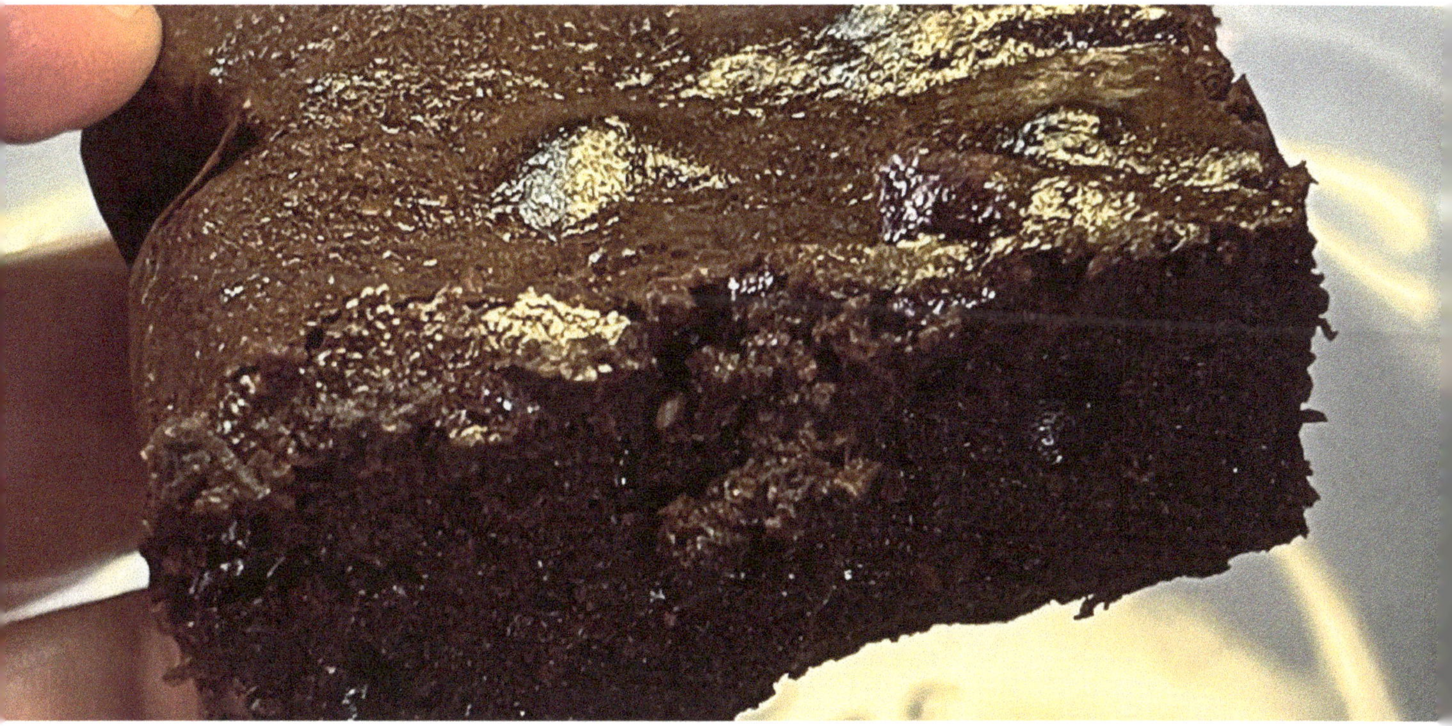

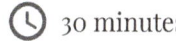 9 servings 30 minutes

INGREDIENTS

- 6 Tbsp coconut oil or ghee
- 1 cup date syrup
- ¾ cup unsweetened cocoa powder
- 3 large eggs, room temperature
- 2 tsp vanilla extract
- 2 tsp brewed coffee, or ½ tsp instant coffee dissolved in 1 Tbsp hot water (optional, boosts chocolate flavor)
- ½ cup almond flour
- ¼ cup tapioca flour
- ½ tsp salt

DIRECTIONS

1. In a medium saucepan over low heat, melt the coconut oil or ghee. Remove from heat and stir in the date syrup and cocoa powder until smooth.
2. In a mixing bowl, beat the eggs, vanilla, and coffee (if using) until combined. Slowly add the chocolate mixture while whisking.
3. Stir in almond flour, tapioca flour, and salt. Mix just until smooth. Batter will be thick.
4. Line an 8×8-inch pan with parchment paper. Pour in batter and smooth the top. Bake at 350°F for 20–25 minutes. A toothpick should come out with moist crumbs, not wet batter.
5. Let cool at least 30–45 minutes for the crackly top to set. Slice into squares. They get even richer and fudgier when stored in the refrigerator.

For extra richness, stir in ⅓ cup unsweetened chocolate chips (like Pascha) and sprinkle a few more on top before baking. Let the brownies cool completely before slicing for the best texture.

BANANA OR PINEAPPLE ICE CREAM
MADE IN THE NINJA CREAMI ICE CREAM MACHINE

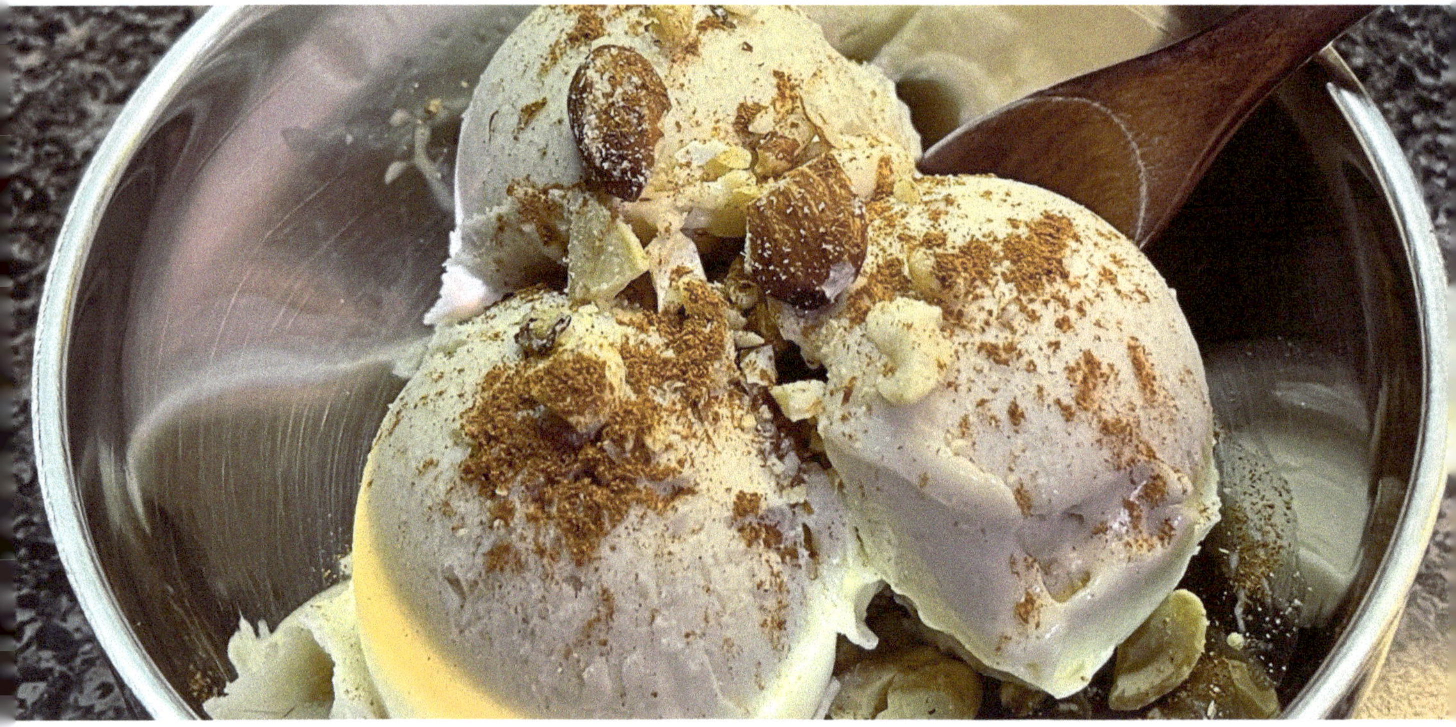

 4 servings 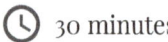 30 minutes

INGREDIENTS

- 1 can (20 oz) crushed pineapple in its own juice, drained, OR
- 2–4 ripe bananas, mashed
- Almond or coconut milk, for re-spinning if needed

DIRECTIONS

1. Add the crushed pineapple or mashed bananas to a Ninja Creami pint container.
2. Freeze for at least 24 hours until solid.
3. When ready, remove the container from the freezer. Insert it into the outer bowl, attach the paddle lid, and lock it into the Ninja Creami machine.
4. Press Power, select Full, then Lite Ice Cream, and press Start.
5. If the texture is crumbly, use the Re-spin function and add a splash of almond or coconut milk for a creamier result.
6. Serve immediately and enjoy.

Nothing makes ice cream this simple like the Ninja Creami. It's worth the investment for how flexible and easy it makes creating healthy frozen treats with just one ingredient.

CHOCOLATE PUDDING

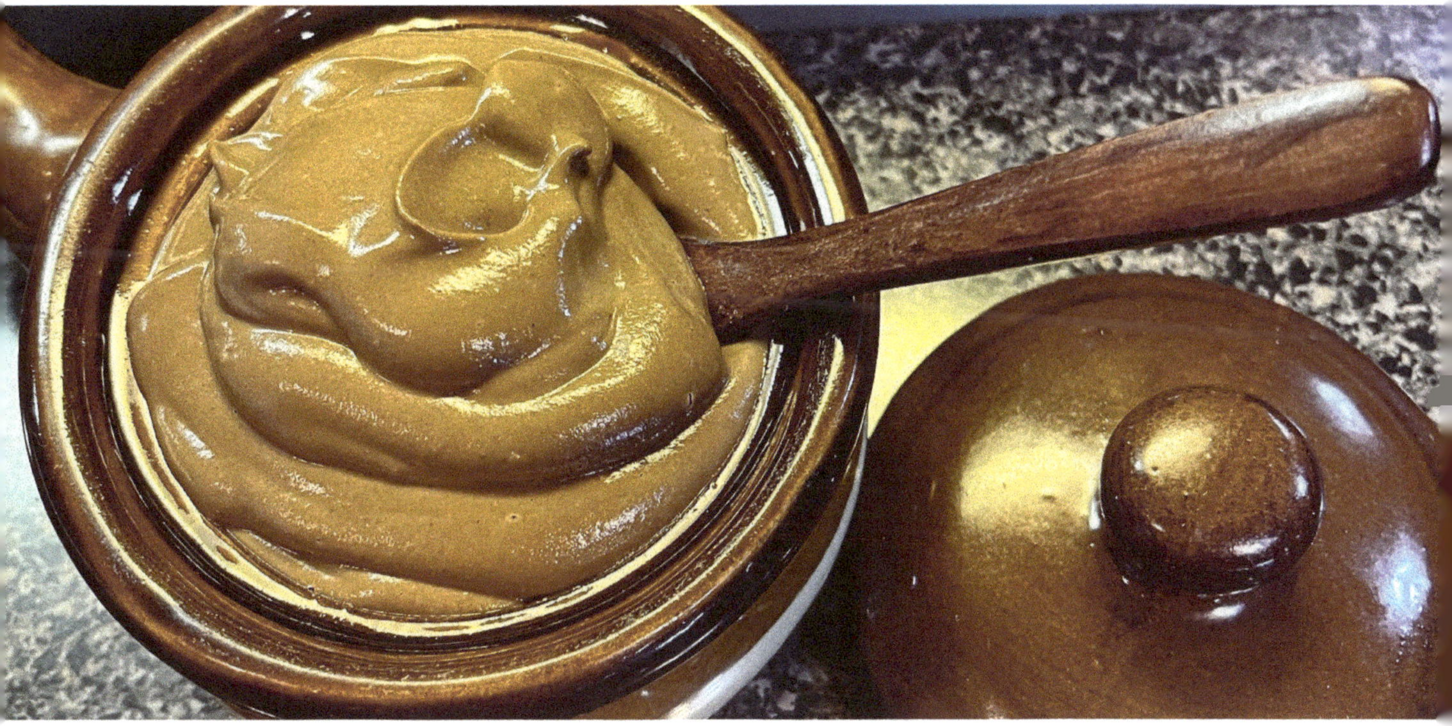

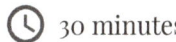

4 servings   30 minutes

INGREDIENTS

- 2 large or 3 small ripe avocados
- ¼ cup coconut cream (the thick part from a chilled can)
- ¼ cup unsweetened cocoa powder
- 2–3 Tbsp almond butter
- 2–4 Tbsp date syrup, to taste
- 1½ tsp vanilla extract
- ⅛ tsp salt, adjusting to taste
- 2–4 Tbsp almond or coconut milk, as needed for blending

DIRECTIONS

1. Add all ingredients to a blender or food processor.
2. Blend until smooth and creamy, scraping down the sides as needed.
3. If it's too thick, blend in almond or coconut milk 1 Tbsp at a time until it reaches a pudding-like texture.
4. Add more date syrup for sweetness, or salt to balance the flavor. Chill for at least 30 minutes before serving.

Serving Ideas
- Top with crushed nuts, toasted coconut, or whipped coconut cream.
- Layer with berries or use as a parfait base.
- Serve with fresh apple slices or strawberries for dipping.

This pudding is rich and versatile—let it chill for at least 30 minutes before serving for the best texture. It also makes a great make-ahead dessert for easy, healthy indulgence!

DUBAI LUXE CHOCOLATE BOWL

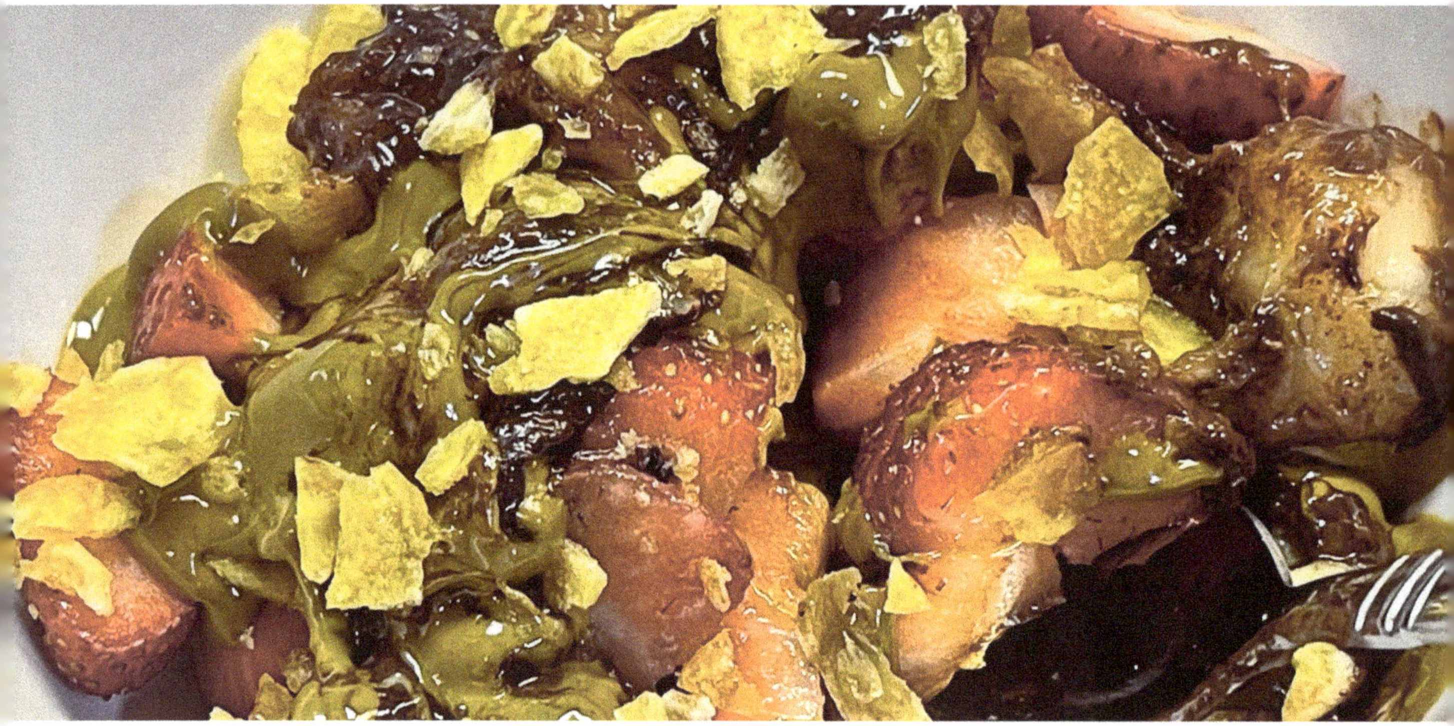

 2 servings 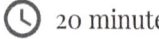 20 minutes

INGREDIENTS

- 1 ripe banana, sliced
- 1 pinch cinnamon
- Small pinch of salt (optional, for balance)
- 1 tsp coconut oil, for frying
- ½ cup fresh strawberries, sliced
- Handful of plantain chips, crushed, plus more for topping
- 1–2 Tbsp pistachio paste, store-bought or homemade
- Optional: 1–2 Tbsp unsweetened chocolate chips, such as Pascha

DIRECTIONS

1. In a serving bowl, layer sliced strawberries as the base.
2. Top strawberries with crushed plantain chips.
3. Heat a small skillet over medium heat and add coconut oil.
4. Fry banana slices in the coconut oil with cinnamon and an optional pinch of salt until caramelized and golden brown, about 2–3 minutes per side.
5. If using, add chocolate chips to the skillet and gently stir to melt and coat the bananas.
6. Spoon the warm banana-chocolate mixture over the strawberry and chip layer.
7. Drizzle pistachio paste over the top.
8. Finish with an extra sprinkle of crushed plantain chips for added crunch.
9. Serve immediately and enjoy warm.

Inspired by Dubai's rich chocolate flavors, this dessert is sweet, layered in texture, and just a touch luxurious. Comfort food with a jewel-toned flair.

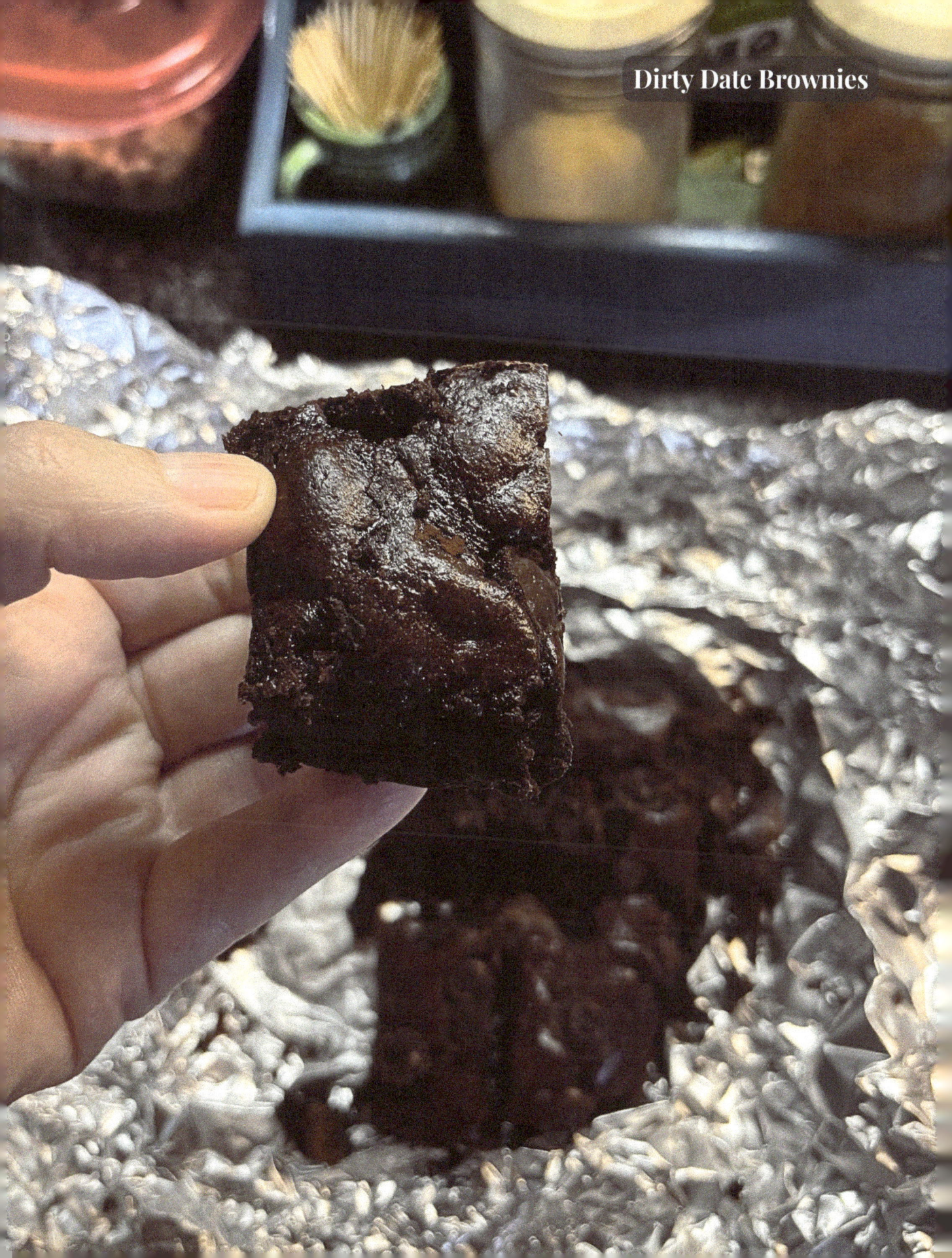

Dirty Date Brownies

WHAT ABOUT BREAKFAST & LUNCH?

I kept this cookbook focused on dinner because that's what made the biggest difference for me. Dinner grounded the day, fed the family, and helped me stay consistent without overthinking everything.

Of course, I also ate breakfast and lunch too. They just weren't fancy. Most mornings, I had things like eggs, RX Bars, coffee with Nutpods unsweetened creamer, or leftovers. Lunch was usually leftover dinner, chicken salad, fruit, or something I could throw together fast.

It wasn't about perfection. It was about feeding myself with what I had and keeping it simple.

You don't need perfection on your plate. Just feed yourself. That's it.

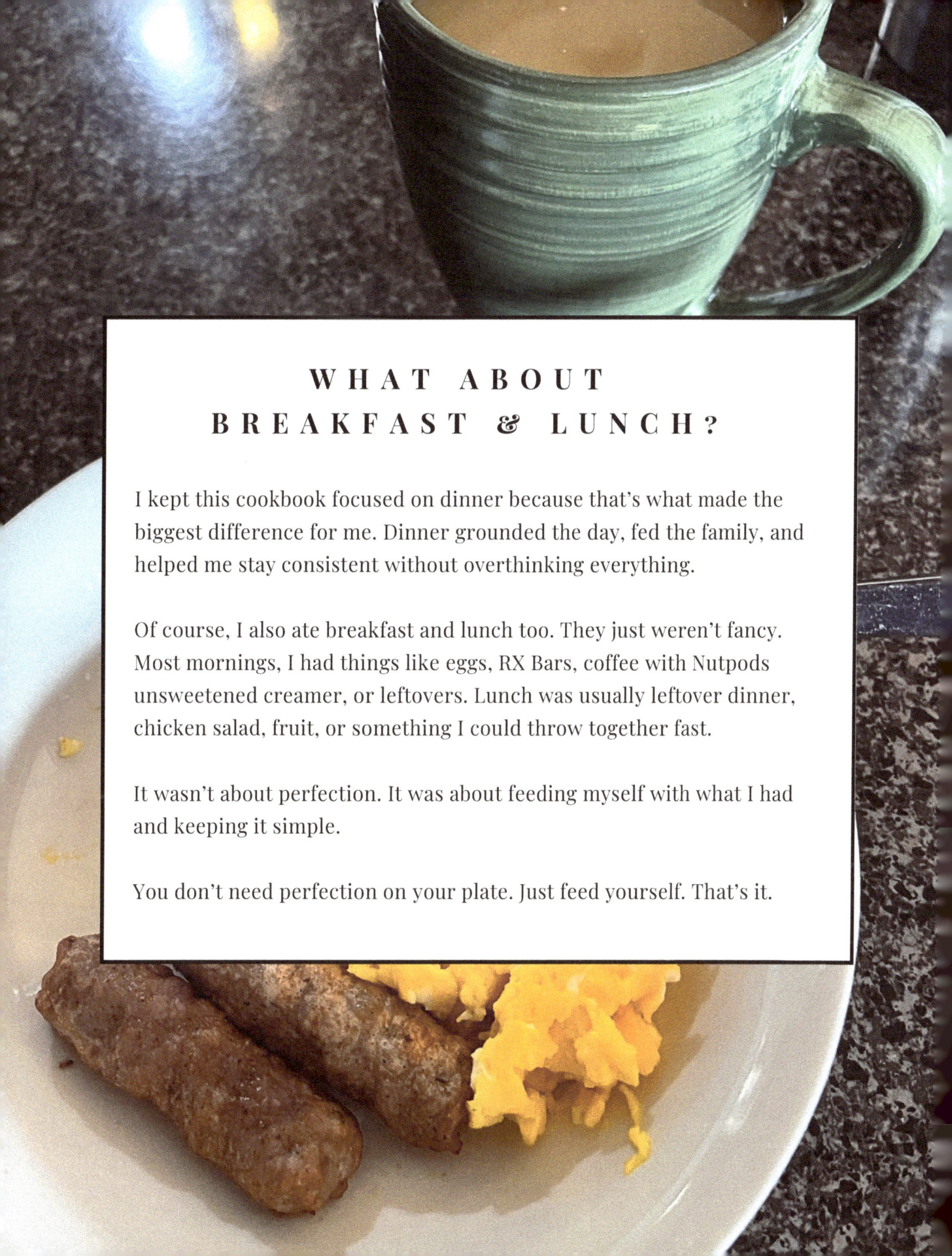

AFTER THE DIRTY RESET

After the Dirty Reset™, I didn't just go back to how I used to eat. But I didn't stay perfectly Dirty either. I just kept what worked.

Some days, that meant adding in other real, comforting foods like rice, beans, or homemade crusty bread baked in my own oven. Not to start over or follow a plan, but just because they help me feel good. That's what mattered.

The Dirty Reset gave me a foundation. It reminded me that I can feed myself and my family in a way that felt better, with more energy, less stress, and food we actually enjoyed. That didn't have to stop at 30 days.

There was no timeline. No food rules. Just an invitation to keep what worked and make room for more of what felt good. One meal at a time.

You saw what worked for me. Now it's your turn. Take what you loved, leave what you didn't, and build your own version of a reset that fits your real life. Whether you cook all 30 dinners or just one, I hope this helps you feel a little more grounded, a little more capable, and a lot more fed.

Until next time, keep it Dirty your way with dinners that are delicious and totally yours. Because real life isn't always clean.

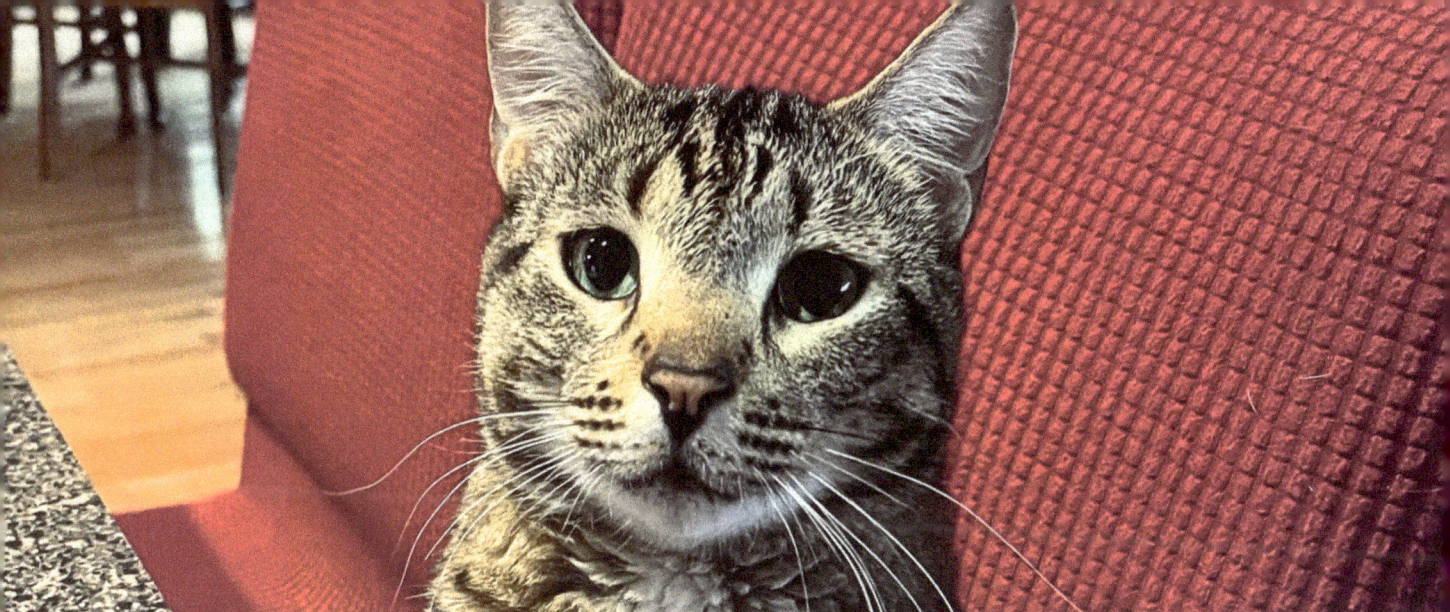

ACKNOWLEDGMENTS

This cookbook is a true DIY. From the words to the recipes to the photos, everything was created with love in my own kitchen, sometimes with Rampage cheering me on.

All recipes, recipe testing, writing, photography, food styling, editing, layout, design, branding, proofreading, and marketing were done by me. Whew! I've been busy. Every effort was made to proofread this book with care, but if a little error slipped through, thank you for your understanding.

ABOUT THE AUTHOR

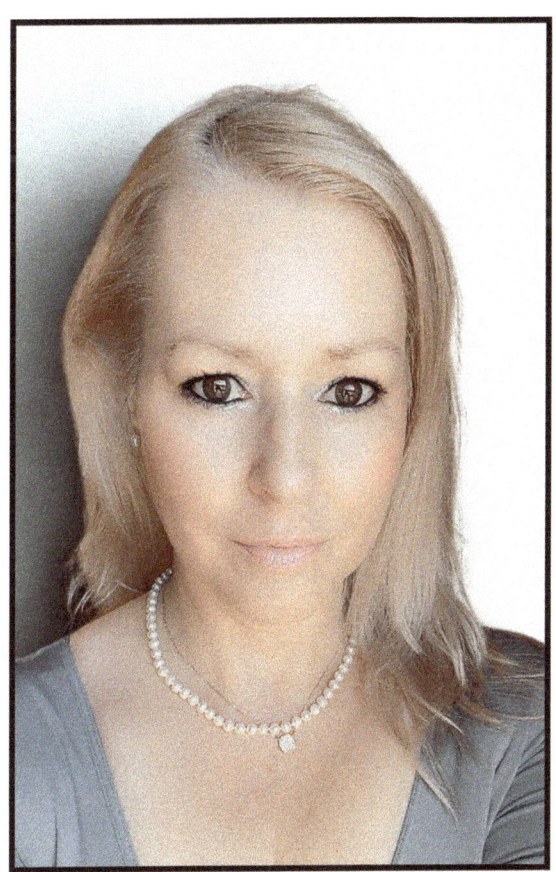

For more recipes, extras, and updates,
head to TheDirtyReset.com.
30 days. My way.
No perfection required.

Wendy Littrell is the creator of The Dirty Reset™, a realistic approach to home cooking built on simple, whole-food meals, flexible habits, and no guilt. She believes food should feel good, taste good, and work in real life.

Her creativity extends beyond the kitchen. From the first time she read *The Giving Tree* by Shel Silverstein and *Too Much Noise* by Ann McGovern as a child, to discovering *Hope for the Flowers* by Trina Paulus as an adult, Wendy has been inspired to create stories that speak to both the young and the young at heart. She has written and self-published several children's books, pairing her words with her own amateur illustrations in the hope of inspiring curiosity and joy in young readers. Through these stories, she highlights the interconnectedness we share and the small meanings that bring us all together.

She is also an avid collector and co-creator of CollectIconic with her husband, where they share their love for pop culture, horror, anime, sci-fi, and all things nostalgic. Whether she's curating a shelf, stirring something in a cast iron pan, or sketching the beginnings of a story, Wendy brings heart, humor, and real-life creativity to everything she shares, including on Facebook and YouTube @CollectIconic and Instagram @CollectIconic_team.

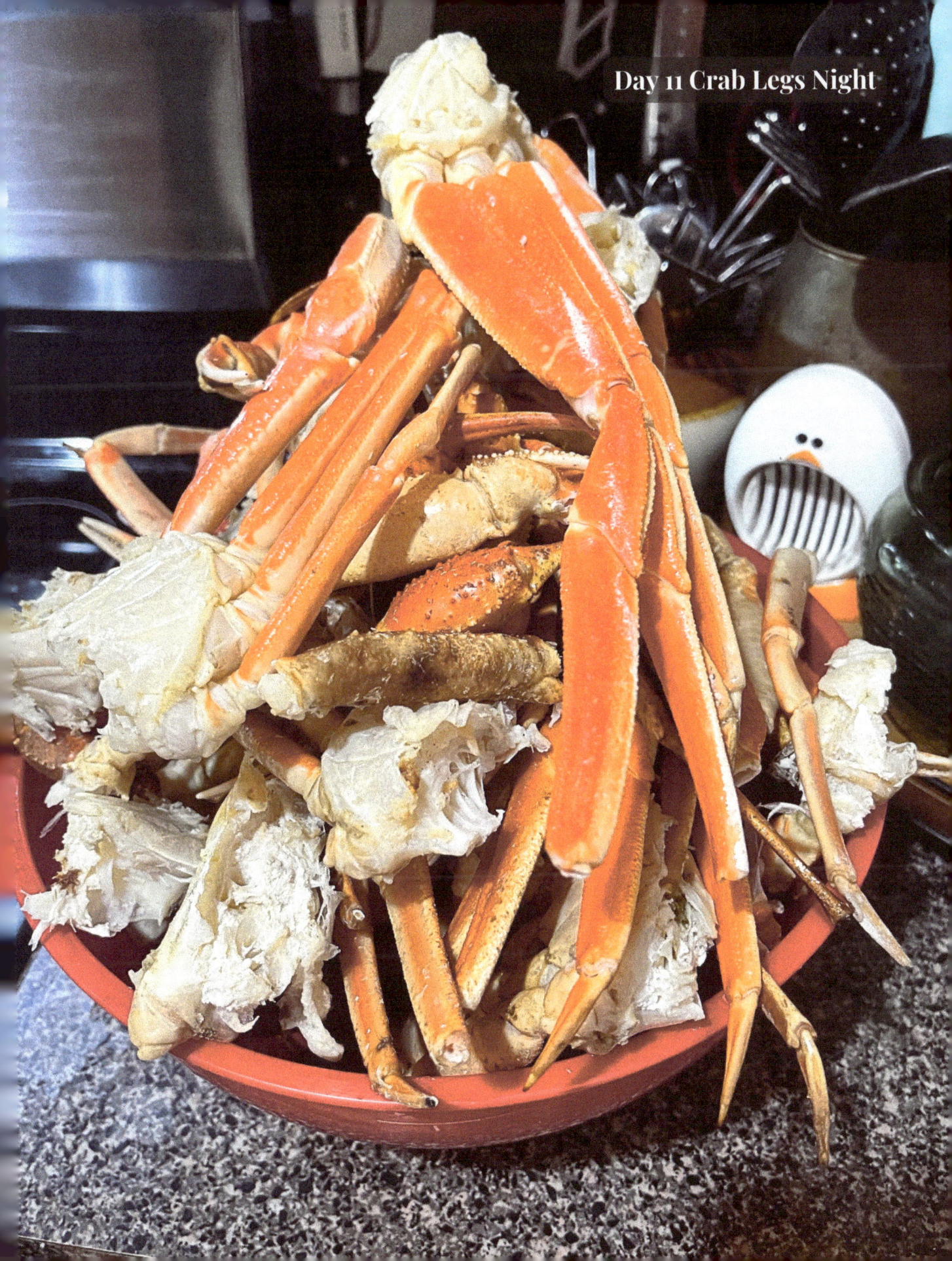

Day 11 Crab Legs Night

this is my kitchen counter